Global health and the new world order

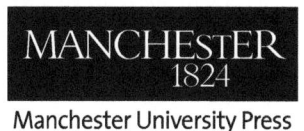
Manchester University Press

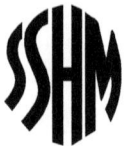

SOCIAL HISTORIES OF MEDICINE

Series editors: *David Cantor, Elaine Leong* and *Keir Waddington*

Social Histories of Medicine is concerned with all aspects of health, illness and medicine, from prehistory to the present, in every part of the world. The series covers the circumstances that promote health or illness, the ways in which people experience and explain such conditions, and what, practically, they do about them. Practitioners of all approaches to health and healing come within its scope, as do their ideas, beliefs, and practices, and the social, economic and cultural contexts in which they operate. Methodologically, the series welcomes relevant studies in social, economic, cultural, and intellectual history, as well as approaches derived from other disciplines in the arts, sciences, social sciences and humanities. The series is a collaboration between Manchester University Press and the Society for the Social History of Medicine.

Previously published

Migrant architects of the NHS *Julian M. Simpson*

Mediterranean quarantines, 1750–1914 Edited by *John Chircop and Francisco Jáviar Martínez*

Sickness, medical welfare and the English poor, 1750–1834 *Steven King*

Medical societies and scientific culture in nineteenth-century Belgium *Joris Vandendriessche*

Vaccinating Britain *Gareth Millward*

Madness on trial *James E. Moran*

Early Modern Ireland and the world of medicine Edited by *John Cunningham*

Feeling the strain *Jill Kirby*

Rhinoplasty and the nose in early modern British medicine and culture *Emily Cock*

Communicating the history of medicine Edited by *Solveig Jülich and Sven Widmalm*

Progress and pathology Edited by *Melissa Dickson, Emilie Taylor-Brown and Sally Shuttleworth*

Balancing the self Edited by *Mark Jackson and Martin D. Moore*

Global health and the new world order

Historical and anthropological approaches to a changing regime of governance

Edited by Jean-Paul Gaudilliere, Claire Beaudevin, Christoph Gradmann, Anne M. Lovell and Laurent Pordié

Manchester University Press

Copyright © Manchester University Press 2020

While copyright in the volume as a whole is vested in Manchester University Press, copyright in individual chapters belongs to their respective authors, and no chapter may be reproduced wholly or in part without the express permission in writing of both author and publisher.

Published by Manchester University Press
Altrincham Street, Manchester M1 7JA

www.manchesteruniversitypress.co.uk

An electronic version of chapter 7 is also available under a Creative Commons (CC-BY-NC-ND) licence, thanks to the support of the Wellcome Trust, which permits non-commercial use, distribution and reproduction provided the editor(s), chapter author and Manchester University Press are fully cited and no modifications or adaptations are made. Details of the licence can be viewed at https://creativecommons.org/licenses/by-nc-nd/4.0/

British Library Cataloguing-in-Publication Data
A catalogue record for this book is available from the British Library

ISBN   978 1 5261 4967 1   hardback

First published 2020

The publisher has no responsibility for the persistence or accuracy of URLs for any external or third-party internet websites referred to in this book, and does not guarantee that any content on such websites is, or will remain, accurate or appropriate.

Typeset
by New Best-set Typesetters Ltd

Contents

List of contributors	*page* vii
Acknowledgements	xi
List of abbreviations	xii

1 Global health and the new world order: introduction 1
   Claire Beaudevin, Jean-Paul Gaudillière,
   Christoph Gradmann, Anne M. Lovell and
   Laurent Pordié

2 Standardization and localization in tuberculosis control 29
   Nora Engel

3 The not-so-distant past, tuberculosis and the DOTS
   challenge 52
   Jean-Paul Gaudillière, Christoph Gradmann and
   Andrew McDowell

4 Decolonizing, nationalizing and globalizing the history
   of psychiatry: from colonial to cross-cultural psychiatry
   in Nigeria 81
   Matthew M. Heaton

5 'Clearing the streets': enacting human rights in mental
   health care in Ghana 103
   Ursula M. Read

6   You've got the point? Acupuncture and the techno-politics
    of bodyscape   130
    Wen-Hua Kuo

7   Finding the global in the local: constructing population
    in the search for disease genes   154
    Steve Sturdy

8   Rare genetic disease, global health and genomics: the
    case of R337h in Brazil   183
    Sahra Gibbon

9   The World Health Organization's response to Ebola in
    historical perspective   207
    Nitsan Chorev

10 Epilogue: in search of global health   230
    Didier Fassin

Index   247

Contributors

Claire Beaudevin is a medical anthropologist and a Tenured Researcher with the French National Centre for Scientific Research (CNRS) at the Cermes3 in Paris. Her current research focuses on the anthropology of genomics and medical genetics in the context of global health. Her main fieldwork is located in the Arabian Peninsula (Sultanate of Oman), where she studies the development of genetics and genomics within the clinic, public health and research. In France, with Catherine Bourgain and Ashveen Peerbaye, she also investigates the development of routine oncogenomics in public hospitals. She recently published: Beaudevin, C., A. Peerbaye and C. Bourgain, 'It has to become true genetics. Tumor genetics and the division of diagnostic labor in the clinic', *Sociology of Health & Illness* 41 (4): 643–657, doi : 10.1111/1467-9566.12844.

Nitsan Chorev is Harmon Family Professor of Sociology and International Studies at Brown University. She specializes in the politics of globalization and neoliberalism, global health and foreign aid. Her second book, *The World Health Organization between North and South* (Cornell University Press, 2012) looked at the transformation of international health policies from the 1970s to the present. Her present research looks at local drug manufacturing in Kenya, Tanzania and Uganda, from the early 1980s onward, to understand the impact of foreign aid on industrial development.

Nora Engel is an assistant professor, Global Health, with the Department of Health, Ethics and Society at Maastricht University. Her research interests lie at the intersection of science and technology, innovation, global health and development. She is the author of *Tuberculosis in India: A Case of Innovation and Control* (Orient Black Swan, 2015).

Didier Fassin is James D. Wolfensohn Professor at the Institute of Advanced Study in Princeton, and Director of studies at the École des Hautes Études en Sciences Sociales. Currently Chair of Public Health at the Collège de France, he has conducted fieldwork in Senegal, Ecuador, South Africa and France. His research explores contemporary political and moral issues. His recent books include *Prison Worlds: An Ethnography of the Carceral Condition* (2016); *The Will to Punish* (2018) and *Life. A Critical User's Manual* (2018).

Jean-Paul Gaudillière is historian of science and senior researcher at the Institut National de la Santé et de la Recherche Médicale, Paris. His research explores the history of the life sciences and medicine during the twentieth century. His recent work focuses on the history of pharmaceutical innovation and the uses of drugs, and on the dynamics of health globalization after the Second World War. He is coordinator of the European Research Council (ERC) project *From International to Global: Knowledge, diseases, and the postwar government of health* (GlobHealth).

Sahra Gibbon is Associate Professor in Medical Anthropology at University College London. Her research examines the social and cultural dimensions of biomedicine. She currently examines how and with what consequences the transnational fields of genomic medicine are being translated in diverse cultural arenas at the interface with the politics and practice of public health care in Latin America. She is the author of *Breast Cancer Genes and the Gendering of Knowledge* (Palgrave Macmillan, 2007).

Christoph Gradmann is Professor of History of Medicine at the Department of Community Medicine and Global Health, University of Oslo. His research mainly focuses on the history of infectious disease in modernity, with, recently, a strong interest in what had happened to infectious diseases when they seemed to be returning at the end of the twentieth century. He is the author of *Laboratory Disease: Robert Koch's Medical Bacteriology* (Johns Hopkins University Press 2009) and co-coordinator of the ERC *GlobHealth* project.

Matthew M. Heaton is an associate professor of History at Virginia Tech. His research focuses on African studies, globalization, health and migration. He has published extensively on the history of Nigeria and is the author of *Black Skin, White Coats: Nigerian Psychiatrists, Decolonization, and the Globalization of Psychiatry* (Ohio University Press, 2013).

Wen-Hua Kuo is Professor of Science, Technology and Society studies at National Yangming University (Tapei), Institute of Public Health. His research the making of modern medicine in non-Western societies. He looks at the globalization of medicine and its impact on East Asia from three aspects: clinical trials at transnational scale, politics of public health, and the transformation of medical professions. He is editor in chief of *East Asian Science, Technology and Society: An International Journal (EASTS)*.

Anne M. Lovell, a medical anthropologist (PhD Columbia University), is Senior Research Scientist Emerita at France's national health institute (INSERM) at CERMES, where she directed the ERC *GlobHealth* project's mental health component. She has studied the social nexus of madness in the US, France, Italy and Senegal. Recent publications include the special issue, 'Genealogies and Anthropologies of Global Mental Health' (*Culture, Medicine and Psychiatry*).

Andrew McDowell is an anthropologist and assistant professor at Tulane University. His research focuses on tuberculosis and tuberculosis control initiatives in India to trace the use by and effects of global health on social science's analytic concepts. As a postdoctoral research fellow in the ERC *GlobHealth* project he conducted an anthropological history of tuberculosis forms and care and their articulation with control policies in India.

Laurent Pordié is an anthropologist specialized in the social study of science and medicine. A Senior Researcher with the National Center for Scientific Research (CNRS) at the CERMES3 (CNRS/EHESS/Inserm) in Paris, he currently works on distribution networks, pharmaceutical regulation and heterodox practices of drug combination in Cambodia. His has recently co-edited *Circulation and Governance of Asian Medicine* (Routledge, 2020).

Ursula M. Read is an anthropologist and research fellow at King's College London in the Department of Global Health and Social Medicine. Since 2005 she has conducted extensive fieldwork in Ghana and published on the impact of mental illness on family life, moral and ethical dilemmas around care and consent, and the relationship between psychiatric services and traditional and faith healers.

Steve Sturdy is Professor of the Sociology of Medical Knowledge at the University of Edinburgh and co-director of the Centre for Biomedicine, Self and Society. His work focuses on the development of medical knowledge and medical practice. He is currently researching the development of 'biomedicine' from the mid-twentieth century to the present, with a particular focus on medical genetics and genomics. He edited with Richard Freeman *Knowledge in Policy: Embodied, Inscribed, Enacted* (Policy Press, 2014).

Acknowledgements

The preparation of this collective volume was made possible by the ERC funding of the project *From International to Global: Knowledge, Disease and the Post-war Government of Health* (Advanced Grant 340510) coordinated by Jean-Paul Gaudillière (Cermes3, Paris) and Christoph Gradmann (University of Oslo). Preliminary versions of some chapters were presented during the inaugural conference of the project, which took place in January 2014.

Abbreviations

CEPH	Centre d'Etude du Polymorphisme Humain
DOTS	Directly Observed Treatment, short course
GBD	Global Burden of Disease
H3Africa	Human Heredity and Health in Africa
HRW	Human Rights Watch
IUATLD	International Union Against Tuberculosis and Lung Disease
MDR-TB	multi-drug resistant tuberculosis
MRC	Medical Research Council
NGO	non-governmental organization
NHGRI	National Human Genome Research Institute
NTI	National Tuberculosis Institute
NTLP	National TB and Leprosy Program
NTP	National Tuberculosis Program
PRC	People's Republic of China
RFLP	restriction fragment length polymorphism
RNTCP	Revised National Tuberculosis Control Programme
SNP	single nucleotide polymorphism
STS	Science, Technology and Society
TB	tuberculosis
TCM	traditional Chinese medicine
UN	United Nations
UNICEF	United Nations Children's Fund
US	United States
WHO	World Health Organization
WPRO	Western Pacific Region Office

1

Global health and the new world order: introduction

Claire Beaudevin, Jean-Paul Gaudillière, Christoph Gradmann, Anne M. Lovell and Laurent Pordié

The phrase 'global health' appears ubiquitously in contemporary medical spheres, from academic research programmes to websites of pharmaceutical companies. In its most visible manifestation, global health refers to strategies addressing major epidemics and endemic conditions through philanthropy (e.g. the Bill and Melinda Gates Foundation) and multilateral, public-private partnerships (e.g. the Global Fund against AIDS, Tuberculosis and Malaria). Within this context, global health can be understood as a series of concerted responses to the perceived failure of decades-long struggles against major infectious diseases in non-industrialized countries, culminating in the post-Second World War era of international health and development. Global health efforts appeal for action in favour of 'neglected' populations by focusing on access to innovative and existing treatments, particularly drugs.

More recently, the scope of global health has expanded to include non-communicable diseases, including psychiatric and neurological conditions, injuries, cardiovascular disease and cancer, as well as innovative screening and treatments, such as medical genetics. In all areas, global health carries a series of assumptions – from the primacy of metrics and evidence-based practices to the incorporation of human-rights and poverty-eradication principles – that seem to oppose the earlier era of international health and development.

This volume moves beyond acknowledgements of the discursive prominence of global health to examine deep transformations regarding the actors, the targets and the tools involved in the governance of health at the international level. We argue not only that the global health enterprise signals a significant departure from the post-war targets and modes of operation that were typical of international public health (1940s–80s) but also that new configurations of action have moved it beyond concerns with infectious diseases and state-based programmes.

Governing health worldwide: history, anthropology and the problem of transition

Global health is of course not meant to be the birth of a governance of health at the international level. Historians have discussed previous waves of health globalization with various ideas about their dynamics and periodization. If the circulation of people, germs and remedies is taken as the main feature, global stories of health often start with the Early Modern period and the colonization of the Americas. In contrast, when considering the existence of institutions, programmes and tools to intervene on the health of others, then the late nineteenth century and the climax of European colonization come to the fore. Rather than focusing on the legacies of these early phases, this volume investigates the relationship of global health to a third wave of health globalization, namely the era of international public health and the regime of health governance that dominated the second half of the twentieth century.

The first use of the term 'global health', according to a Pubmed database search, appears in the 1940s, but the expression does not really become frequent until the 1980s. By 2015, over 20,000 articles concerned with global health could be identified through the Web of Science. One interpretation of this growth may be that the term itself serves as what sociologists of science call a boundary object, linking heterogeneous and novel forms of knowledge, practices and actors involved in health interventions at a worldwide level (Weisz et al., 2017). This view of global health as a marker of recent and large transformations in the governance of health at the international level is not really new. Both historians and anthropologists of medicine have addressed the changes of the late twentieth century, although in very contrasting ways.

To remind us of what we owe to the former, one may recall the classic 2006 paper by Brown, Cueto and Fee from their project on the history of the World Health Organization (WHO) (Brown et al., 2006). In their paper global health is – to a large extent – a political phenomenon placed in the context of geopolitics, development strategies and rivalry between international organizations. Focusing on the WHO and the United Nations (UN) system of intergovernmental democracy, they point to the intimate relationship that international public health maintained with the Cold War. Other authors like Birn (2009) and Chorev (2012), as well as Cueto, Brown and Fee in their recent monograph (2019), have operated within comparable framings. Similarly, Packard, in his monograph (2016), has argued for more long-term continuity but seems to confirm the centrality of the 1980s–2000s as a period of change. To the historian, global health appears as both response and adaptation to a new situation dominated by a neoliberal agenda, associated with the rise of the World Bank alongside (and sometimes displacing) the WHO in the area of health, the quantification of health as an economic factor, the generalization of public-private partnerships and alliances independent from the UN system and the call for mobilizing 'civil society' rather than nation-states.

Anthropologists bring a different perspective to this transition, by stressing heterogeneity within global health and the specificities of local realities. One of the most widely read ethnographies of global health, Julie Livingston's monograph on the only cancer ward in Botswana, illustrates this approach (Livingston, 2012). The improvised medicine which she describes challenges notions of universality by revealing global health to be a matter of practices under constraint. Oncology at the periphery, as opposed to, say, in New York, inevitably involves a cancer epidemic, which does not fit the global agenda of oncology research and treatment. The nature of this epidemic challenges the once-dominant idea of an epidemiological transition from infectious to chronic disease according to which low-income countries would eventually exhibit the same patterns found earlier in the industrialized North. Cancer cases in Botswana tend to develop from almost-forgotten viruses and are often poly-morbid with AIDS and tuberculosis (TB). Furthermore, patients exhibit critical advanced stages of the disease rarely seen in wealthier settings.

Yet, this oncology at the periphery is simultaneously global. In Botswana as in many places in Africa, the 1980s–90s turn away from international health and development was less about new responses than the destruction of old ones. The debt crisis and structural adjustment policies, with their parade of reduced public funding for health, tightening cost management and experimental introduction of patients' fees, have left deep traces on an already ruined landscape that resonates with historical studies. The global percolates into the local with new forms of circulation linked to drug access, the interventions of public-private partnerships and philanthropic actors, from the Bill and Melinda Gates Foundation to pharmaceutical companies like Novartis.

What is at stake here is not the incompatibility of such historical and anthropological approaches. On the contrary, their combination has generated important insights in recent historical work about global health, for instance in explorations of medical experiments in East Africa (Graboyes, 2015), of mass therapeutic campaigns in French colonial Africa (Lachenal, 2014; Tousignant, 2012) or of the vestiges of medical research in West and East Africa (Geissler et al., 2016). Several anthropologists have also recently combined ethnographies of globalized health with historical approaches when attending, for instance, to HIV/AIDS, leprosy and malaria in Africa (Geissler, 2015), to traditional healing and its role in Tanzania (Langwick, 2015) or to the meaning of past 'African science' in a Ghanaian laboratory (Droney, 2014). However, this scholarship is characterized both by its scarcity and by its predominantly African focus, where historians and anthropologists have long and parallel experience in using oral histories.

As a consequence, the prevailing disconnection between historical and anthropological approaches in studies of international/global health has created a vast body of literature and two formidable gaps. The first is a temporal gap between the historiography of international public health through the 1970s and the numerous anthropological studies of global health in the present. In between the two periods lies the far less commonly analysed transition beginning in the 1980s–2000s. The second gap originates in problems of scale. Macro-inquiries of institutions and politics abound, as do micro-investigations of local configurations. Taken together, they omit intermediate spaces through which these levels might be linked, such as local and regional non-governmental organizations (NGOs), as well as objects and actors that circulate: experts, pharmaceuticals, tools and policies. With this book we contribute to filling these gaps through a stronger engagement between history and anthropology, an attention to the history of the present and a harnessing of concepts (circulation, scale, transnationalism) that cross the two disciplines.

Bringing historians and anthropologists into a closer conversation, at times based on integrated research, the book thus allows knowledge, practices and policies to be linked, while bridging the macro-history of post-war international health and the local anthropology of the present. We identify crucial and differentiated moments in the postwar trajectory of transnational health interventions. We define them in terms of diseases targeted, actors involved, expertise mobilized, tools employed and – given their importance in the turn to global – the relations between health, development and economy. The periodization, in which a sea-change occurs between the mid-1980s and the late 1990s, rests on our hypothesis that multiple practices of health globalization were already in existence by, or first appeared at, the end of the Second World War. The consequence is that one can, for analytical purposes, conceptualize two different regimes or ways of 'doing health' outside Europe and North America: the regime of international public health, which dominated the first four decades of the post-war era; and the regime of global health, which has gradually stabilized since the turn of the century.

Within the regime of international public health, control of selected infectious diseases, especially smallpox and malaria, dominated the agenda (Bhattacharya, 2006; Cueto, 2007; Howard-Jones, 1981; Lee, 2009). The WHO and other intergovernmental bodies initiated and prioritized eradication campaigns. Eradication, major actors thought, was a technological problem to be dealt with through standardization, expert evaluation of needs and benefits, and centralization of investments and action. UN agencies and major United States (US) foundations coordinated these programmes by defining the targets, delivering the means of intervention and providing some of the infrastructure (notably vaccines for smallpox and insecticides for malaria). During this first period, drugs and clinical care played a role that was secondary to prevention strategies, which mobilized vaccines as well as social control techniques in the fight against infectious diseases. These programmes appeared critical to the reconstruction of post-war Europe as well as for the stabilization of African and Asian colonies (Staples, 2006).

This landscape started to shift in the 1960s, partly as a result of two major changes: on the one hand, the new socio-political climate, associated with the Cold War and the East–West divide, and on the other hand, the decolonization and emergence of numerous new nation-states whose economic, social and political life focused on the 'need for development' (Sidiqi, 1995; Amrith, 2006). This shift also stemmed from the emergence of biomedicine as the dominant form of medical knowledge. It became the basis upon which a rapid expansion of therapeutic tools could be envisioned as a driver of modernization. This period included the massive expansion of the pharmaceutical industry through both its research and development capacities and the consumption of chemotherapeutics, in the US and eastern and western Europe (Dumit, 2012; Gaudillière and Hess, 2013; Gaudillière and Thoms, 2015; Greene, 2007). Echoing mounting legal and administrative regulation in nation-states, the international health agenda began addressing the question of clinical evaluation, toxicology and detection of adverse effects. An additional dimension of this 'drug and development' regime was the rising interest in chronic diseases, fuelled by the idea of an epidemiological as well as a demographic transition or stage of development supposedly realized (in the North) and sought for (in the South).

The significant turning point of the 1970s corresponded to the opening up of official international spaces in which international public health and its programmes were reframed. The Alma-Ata conference organized by the WHO in 1978 is a well-known event linked to the context of decolonization and the mounting influence of a self-defined 'Third World'. Criticism of eradication programmes (Lee, 1997; Litsios, 1997; Webb, 2008) and of the failure of earlier biomedical technologies to meet the needs of the poorest populations brought to the fore a call for the integration of health and social policies, simpler technologies and primary health care as a response to the most basic of medical needs. Renewed interests in 'social health' were translated not only into central and local initiatives to provide access to 'essential' therapies but also into discourses and projects for 'modernizing', 'rationalizing' and 'integrating' traditional medicines.

Around 1990 the end of the Cold War and the emergent neoliberal phase of economic globalization had not only undermined the 'Third World' coalition and the centrality of the WHO but also provided an alternate model of development focused on liberalization policies, minimal state involvement, civil society empowerment and high-tech investment (Petryna, 2009; Petryna et al., 2006). This model remains the core of contemporary global health. It percolated into health policies through an increasing emphasis on local and capacity-building initiatives, individual choices and risk management. A multiplicity of actors ranging from the World Bank to charitable foundations like the Global Fund and a myriad of health- and community-related NGOs effected these changes (Muraskin, 2005; Page, 2007; Rao, 1999). Interests in risk epidemiology and biotechnology strengthened the importance of chronic disorders as global rather than simply Northern or post-development problems, as well as of obesity, mental disorders and genetic diseases. Yet, rather than vanishing, the attention to infectious diseases and epidemics then increased, with the AIDS epidemic, the 'global return' of TB and the resurgence of supposedly new infectious diseases, like viral haemorrhagic fevers. This in turn fuelled new anthropologies of chronic and 'chronicized' disorders (Brown and Kelly, 2014; Farmer and Sen, 2004; Livingston, 2012), controversies about 'neglected' diseases and multiple initiatives to avoid 'market failures': i.e. production of generics, public-private research partnerships and foundation-based distribution programmes (Cassier, 2003; Greene, 2014).

The advent of the Global Burden of Disease (GBD) represents a central marker of the changes wrought in the 1990s. It enables epidemiological-economic assessments applicable to living populations worldwide by focusing on the *absence of health*, now defined not only by excess mortality but by disability as well (Murray and Lopez, 1996). For one, as we discuss below, it renders non-communicable diseases, such as disabling chronic mental illnesses, visible. Like global indices more generally, this new metrics extends globalization through standardization and evaluation beyond infectious disease to the management of risk. The drive for evidence-based practices, coupled with this new 'universal' metrics, opens up new tensions (Adams, 2016).

This scenario goes against the idea of a simple replacement or substitution of one regime by another. As an example, eradication and other vertical programmes typical of the first wave of health internationalization have not disappeared, as historians argue (Packard, 2016). Although the assemblage of actors, tools and targets which they involve profoundly differs from that of the international health era, vertical programmes remain legitimate and central – as the massive presence of HIV, malaria and TB programmes in global health demonstrates.

This volume thus proposes an encompassing view of a historical transition from international public health to global health. Beyond the articulation of history and anthropology two methodological choices allow us to grasp the transition in its profundity: a combined approach that examines actors, targets and tools through in-depth observation and analysis; and the selection of four fields in the globalization of health that we deem illustrative of the range of sectors touched by the globalization of health today: infectious disease (TB), non-communicable disease (mental health), traditional medicine (Asian medicines) and high-technology medical innovations (medical genetics). Within each field, the authors interrogate specific assemblages to approach *processes* rather than structures. While never losing sight of local specificities, the chapters emphasize transversal processes, such as movements of 'localization' and 'generalization' that challenge attempts at making 'things [purely] global' in the name of universality by overriding their situated ontologies.

The return of TB as a worldwide neglected disease

TB provides a paradigmatic example of the changing management of a major infectious disease, from one health regime to another. An infectious disease that has been in the focus of public health for centuries and that used to play an important role in the old nexus between the social and the medical, TB was a major international public health concern until the 1960s. Its multiple causalities have led its treatment to sweep the entire range of therapeutic practices, from isolation to treatment surveillance to drugs. While TB provided the iconic social disease of industrial societies, thus giving priority to institutional treatment and assistance, the Second World War was a turning point (Condrau and Worboys, 2010; McMillen, 2015; Packard, 1989). Under the auspice of UN organizations, specific antibiotic therapies dominated care in developed countries, while BCG vaccination campaigns were framed as a medical strategy of modernization in developing countries. As supplements to control strategies based on vaccination, combination chemotherapies of increasingly shorter duration were designed. Until the 1960s some pharmacological innovation was undertaken, but by the 1970s TB was considered to be on the road to eradication. Lung and respiratory medicine specialists faced a professional crisis, while the WHO put its TB expert committee on hold and effectively suspended its TB programmes.

In contrast to this relatively well-known history, the path which led the WHO to reinstate its programme against tuberculosis in 1995, in response to a resurgence of the disease driven by the HIV epidemic and sustained poverty rates, has barely been explored. Nor has the specific relationship of context to this reinstatement, notably the changing institutional landscape, been explored: the increased interest of the World Bank in efficient health investments as growth factors alongside mounting critiques of the absence and/or the poor performance of TB control programmes in the global South (World Bank, 1993). Several elements – beyond the co-infection of TB and HIV – seem to differentiate the global tuberculosis from the 1990s onwards from TB policy in previous decades. TB is now viewed as 'neglected' in terms both of access to chemotherapeutics and of research investments into drug development. As a threat of global dimensions, it now necessitates standardized tools and integrated and centralized programmes within a global strategy. TB today is also a different disease, multi-drug resistant; and the absence of novel drugs raises major concerns resulting in ongoing monitoring of risks, i.e. of the circulation of strains and the organization of chemotherapy (Kim et al., 2005).

International actors have accordingly implemented different approaches from those of previous programmes. Directly Observed Treatment, short course (DOTS), which became the preferred approach in the early 1990s based on an initiative and trials run by the International Union Against Tuberculosis and Lung Disease (IUATLD), was picked up by the World Bank and implemented through the WHO. It built on the insight that failed control of tuberculosis was less the consequence of misconceived strategies than a problem of poor administration of treatments (Gradmann, 2019). DOTS consists of a whole package of which the therapeutic regimen is only one aspect. The others include political commitment with increased and sustained financing; case detection through quality-assured bacteriology; standardized treatment, with supervision of patients; an effective drugs supply and management system; monitoring, evaluation and impact measurement.

Solutions are therefore to be sought in standardization of tools and protocols, surveillance and control of patients to ensure compliance, good organization and performance assessment (Harper, 2010).

The chapters included in the book thus approach the construction of DOTS, as a standardized 'package' that epitomizes global health in the TB health sector, in two different ways. Based on anthropological fieldwork in India, Nora Engel (chapter 2) explores how DOTS programmes have been standardized, operated and eventually amended in different social contexts. In their contribution in chapter 3, Jean-Paul Gaudillière, Christoph Gradmann and Andrew McDowell combine their historical and anthropological research in Tanzania and India to trace the research and policy initiatives taken by the IUATLD, the WHO and, later, the World Bank. From the late 1970s to the mid-1990s these actions paved the way for DOTS to become the technique considered the single best means of controlling tuberculosis, first in East Africa and later in India, where the DOTS strategy replaced a national programme based on radically different assumptions (Brimnes, 2016).

A global psychiatry? From colonial histories to global mental health

Global mental health presents a contrasting example to the case of TB within the regime of global health, since it is associated with neither large investments nor internationally implemented standards for diagnosis and therapy. Although local variations in disease presentation and management in general trouble assumptions of universality (Livingston, 2012; Lock and Nguyen, 2018), diagnostic classification in mental health is particularly prone to epistemic weakness. Mental disorders suggest clusters, associations and dimensions rather than a bounded 'disease'; and diagnoses must rely on subjective patient report rather than biomarkers. Despite advances in neurosciences and genetics and revisions of the Diagnostic and Statistical Manual (DSM-5) and the behavioural health section of the International Classification of Diseases (ICD-11), the content, structure and appropriateness of categories as psychiatric continue to be debated within psychiatry (Hyman, 2010; Kleinman, 2012; Van Os et al., 2009), anthropology (Kleinman, 2012) and sociology (Horwitz and Wakefield, 2007). Epistemological weakness introduces refractoriness to the mere incorporation of mental health into a global health agenda applicable everywhere.

Mental health was incorporated from the start into the WHO constitution's definition of health. Until the early 1960s WHO's experts and NGO collaborators produced a highly normative, idealist notion of mental health as the capacity to live harmoniously with others (Lovell, 2014). Although the international public health focus on infectious disease marginalized psychiatry, the WHO developed an international psychiatric epidemiology to establish the universality of mental illnesses. Needs created by the dearth of psychiatrists in low-income countries competed with WHO research (Lovell, 2014), undergirded by the post-war 'charm of internationalism' (Wu, 2015).

In a parallel development, the WHO supported racialized research on 'the mind of African man' (Carothers, 1953), eventually debunked through post-colonial psychiatries. Recent historical scholarship enlightens our understanding of these processes, including the post-independence drive for the creation of dedicated institutions. It also moves beyond single-nation (or colony) case studies by focusing on transnational connections, from the circulation of knowledge between centre and periphery (Ernst, 2013) to the social, political and other influences on psychiatric phenomena, such as trauma, treatment and violation of the suffering, beyond the confines of colony or nation-state (e.g. Hunt, 2015; Keller, 2008).

None of these studies, however, allows us to link an earlier period of international (mental) health with the transition towards global mental health. This is precisely the contribution of historian Matthew Heaton in chapter 4. Examining Nigeria, a flagship of burgeoning post-war psychiatry in the newly emerging African nations, Heaton's narrative challenges the diffusion of knowledge from centre to periphery approach. He shows that the circulation of psychiatrists from the global South shaped, at different levels, what would become the treatment and research practices of international psychiatry. The production of epidemiological knowledge in Nigeria during the post-war period reinforced the universality thesis alongside the evidence for patho-plasticity in cultural expressions of mental illnesses. At the same time, the corps of local psychiatrists and their internationally recognized research embodied an intended project of modernity for the new Nigerian state.

Given the epistemological weakness of psychiatry, the impact of the development of GBD metrics, mentioned earlier in this introduction, cannot be overstated. By elaborating a metrics based on disability rather than on mortality alone, GBD analyses could move depression to the top of the 'disease hierarchy' worldwide (Murray and Lopez, 1996). This provided dramatic new visibility for mental health and a new sense of urgency about mental health problems globally (Desjarlais, 1995).

Paradoxically, the reliance on metrics – the data-production and number-crunching dimension of what Vincanne Adams and her colleagues call the global sovereign (Adams, 2016) – strengthens the epistemological assumption of 'thingness', *as if* numbers represented objective substrates. Nevertheless, they raise the question of how psychiatric globalization is materially achieved. Three processes provide illustrations. First, depression is being transformed from a minor psychiatric category focused on clinical severity (i.e. melancholia) into a moderate disorder, widely diagnosed with brief symptom scales and managed by general practitioners and primary health care workers. New frameworks provide continuity with local meaning by incorporating older healing practices and interpretations of distress into new modalities (Behrouzan, 2016; Lang and Jansen, 2013). Second, trauma and the invention of trauma-related diagnoses like Post-Traumatic Stress Disorder (PTSD) (Young, 1997) similarly cast a wide net. This is made possible by the collective re-reading of historical and present-day violence and trauma through the lens of pathology and by the widely diffused therapeutic techniques developed in response to PTSD (Fassin and Rechtman, 2009). Third, psychiatry is ever more concerned with complex though aetiologically uncertain biological aetiologies and associations, despite epistemic blinders (Hyman, 2010). Increased biologization drives pharmaceutical interventions, incorporated into global mental health packages alongside psychosocial techniques.

Recent edited volumes in anthropology focus on cultural and local differences in global mental health (White et al., 2017), but they neither analyse the broader changes identified above nor problematize global mental health (Kohrt and Mendenhall, 2016). Anthropologist Ursula Read's chapter 5 in this book does all three. She presents a hybrid project of human rights within global mental health, defined as an assemblage of statistical tools, equipment, relational and organizational forms, community organizations and human rights guidelines. In Ghana, her fieldwork site, these components comprise non-negligible *devices for governance and governmentality* alongside older, more insidious forms.

Ghana's flagship mental health reforms allow her to explore the implementation of human rights as a core element of global mental health, diffused and monitored by global actors like the WHO, the UN and Human Rights Watch. By combining historical research with anthropology, Read is able to show how this new ethics, appropriated and reformulated to local ends, incorporates traces of practices and frameworks from an older, pre-global health era.

Globalizing therapeutic techniques and industrial products from Asian medicine

From the late 1970s onward, the WHO, states like China and India, as well as local firms and practitioners of Asian medicine, have sought to put the question of the making, evaluation and uses of herbal preparations on the agenda of international health. This seems to have been a huge success: bio-prospection in collaboration with industry still exists in spite of a noticeable decline due to technical difficulties and juridical uncertainty; the protection of traditional knowledge is an object of international negotiations; the markets for mass-produced herbal medicines link Europe, the United States, Asia and Latin America.

Asian medicines are subject to international regulations on production, registration and quality control; they are elements in heterogeneous treatment strategies targeting chronic disorders, juxtaposing biomedical with so-called complementary and alternative therapies. If this dual process of industrialization and broad circulation has remained at the margins of global health as an autonomous field with its specific programmes and sets of institutions, it is nonetheless a crucial development in the globalization of health as powerfully illustrated by the policies of China or India (Alter, 2005; Banerjee, 2009; Bode, 2008; Coderey and Pordié, 2019; Pordié, 2011; Zhan, 2009).

Two contextual layers are therefore important to understand the processes of globalization and industrialization, which seem to presently dominate the transformation of Asian medicines, and their rather peripheral presence in global health when considered at the level of organizations and programmes. The entry of traditional medicine, and especially Asian medicine, into the world health scenario goes back to the 1950s, when the WHO and UNICEF (the UN Children's Fund) decided together to provide biomedical training to healers in the Philippines. This project signalled the beginning of a new era for traditional medicines worldwide, and was influenced by two Asian examples: Chinese medicine and the barefoot doctors, and Indian medical pluralism. However, it was, not until 1975 that the need to integrate traditional therapeutic practices into health care policies was recognized and adopted by the Executive Committee of the WHO, and subsequently by the World Health Assembly in 1977. To simplify a long and tumultuous story, the idea was to bring traditional healers onto the international public health bandwagon, to ensure that their therapeutic techniques and medical treatments were accessible and safe, and, more importantly, to favour integrative medicine by injecting biomedical ideas and practices into traditional medicine. This approach was consolidated by the WHO in the years following the famous Alma-Ata conference of 1978 and became part of the ambitious programme 'Health for All by the Year 2000'. This was an international public health programme.

By 2020 the discourses and programmes of the WHO had taken a decisive turn. The two global strategies (2002 and 2014) of the WHO for traditional medicine remain centred on the problem of efficacy and integrative medicine, but they no longer approach traditional medicines solely from the perspective of endogenous health development, but from an (economically) globalized perspective, in particular by emphasizing the growing demand for natural medicines in the West. This multilateral organization thus supports a phenomenon which is primarily led by the industry, firmly anchored in national and global market construction rather than inscribed in the programmes led by the new global health actors. And indeed, we observe two fundamental additions to the WHO policies: a strong concern with intellectual property rights, on the one hand, and with the practice and pharmaceutical monitoring of Chinese and Asian medicine in the West, on the other hand. Asian medicines are now explicitly part of globalized health practices, not only in economic terms or as sources of future cures but also as direct answers to infectious diseases and epidemics, as the cases of natural antimalarials, or the outbreaks of chikungunya, SARS or avian flu have shown (e.g. Craig and Adams, 2008).

The second layer overlaps these various concerns. The worldwide unification of markets and the generalization of neoliberal regulations and forms of governance have impacted on the pharmaceutical milieu.

In pharmaceutics a new phase in this complex process began with the *Agreement on Trade-Related Aspects of Intellectual Property Rights* (TRIPS), adopted in 1994, which concerns intellectual property rights. This resulted in the international diffusion and recognition of drug patents, initially promoted by the US to put an end to 'pirating' by countries like India and to generate incentives to develop local research that could then be appropriated. Economic reasoning thus plays an essential role in the realm of pharmacy, including 'indigenous pharmacy', but does not explain all the changes engendered by pharmaceutical globalization. Understood less restrictively as a twofold movement – to extend circulation (of commodities, persons or knowledge) and to set up procedures to govern it – globalization has reconfigured relations between the singular and the collective, deeply affecting ways of thinking and of acting in all corners of the world. In pharmaceutical globalization, interconnections reach beyond just market trading. Changes in the world of pharmacy are in fact not only related to trade and intellectual property, they also have to do with standardizing research or production practices (Pordié and Gaudillière, 2014), and also with the requirement to adapt therapeutic practices originating in Asian medicine to the regulatory frameworks of certain Asian, European or North American countries (Pordié, 2014) and to the expectations of practitioners and consumers in those parts of the world, as chapter 6 by Wen-Hua Kuo powerfully shows in the case of acupuncture.

Between research and clinical practice: globalizing genetic and genomic medicine

Since the early twentieth century, from eugenic policies to bioethical debates about genetic screening or the medical promises of national genome projects and gene therapy, medical genetics and genomics have been widely studied by social sciences in the North. Their history is well documented (as detailed by Steve Sturdy in chapter 7), their clinical dimensions are scrutinized and their technological advances and implications are followed. However, medical genetics and genomics are not solely 'Northern phenomena': millions of individuals worldwide are affected by so-called rare disorders, and the related genetic and genomic knowledge and tools circulate in shifting ways to, from and within the global South. Such a scope leaves marks into the main tools and institutions of the global health field: the GBD lists several inherited diseases and the WHO has implemented dedicated programmes (briefly discussed in the following sections). Still, the worldwide expansion of genetic medicine and genomic research in (public) health policy, clinical practice and research did not lead to their inscription in the central categories and targets of global health interventions.

Studying the globalization of genetic and genomic medicine is thus a twofold endeavour which requires simultaneously investigating multiple, non-scaled-up WHO initiatives on medical genetics and the manifold ways in which genes, genomics and related health matters were internationalized, independently of the main global health actors. Genetics and genomics have indeed long gone global, with patients travelling for treatment; DNA samples being placed on board airplanes; scientists, health care professionals and lay individuals sharing genomic data over the web; laboratories buying technologies abroad; genetic counselling being taught transnationally; genetic knowledge taking shape in universities, hospitals and conferences worldwide; new local and global markets for genetic tests blossoming.

The WHO's interest in genetics started in the 1950s and was originally rooted in studies of the impact of radiation on health. Later, it expanded to the investigation of heredity, with large neonatal studies in the 1960s and investigations of isolated (and supposedly primitive) populations (de Chadarevian, 2015; Lindee, 2014). Over the following decades, genetics became increasingly seen as a central part of the effort to acquire health for all, with the WHO's advocacy in the 1980s of community genetics programmes in the wealthiest of its member states (Gaudillière et al., forthcoming; Ruault et al., forthcoming). This call aimed at organizing testing and genetic counselling for common hereditary disorders, as one of the most outstanding examples of the belief in genetics as a public health essential. The community genetics effort chiefly started in Cyprus and expanding subsequently into the Eastern Mediterranean region of the WHO, with experts helping to create screening and counselling programmes for beta-thalassemia (Modell and Kuliev, 1998; WHO, 1981). The Organization then discussed the introduction of genetic services into developing countries in the late 1980s. The increasing mobilization of actors and resources characteristic of global health's lift-off fundamentally affected health infrastructures and the circulation of medical care, technologies, knowledge, moralities and modes of engagement. This profound modification propelled an expansion of medical genetics beyond the global North. In 2005 the WHO issued a policy recommending the worldwide availability of medical genetics in primary health care.

Significant advances in genetic and genomic research – largely related to population genetics as discussed by Steve Sturdy in chapter 7 – occurred around this date, including the milestone of the decoding of the human genome in 2003. The whole field of human genetics, including medical genetics, has considerably benefited from this new knowledge and related techniques, as well as from the new affordability of diagnostic tools. Consequently, genetic testing has become increasingly available in the global South within the framework of reproductive medicine and prenatal diagnosis in relation to hereditary disorders, or in the field of oncogenetics. This expansion has occurred in various ways: mostly in the private sector, such as described, for instance, for cancer in Brazil by Gibbon (2013, 2018); through both in-house genomic laboratories hosted by public hospitals and partnering with foreign private genomic companies such as in Oman (Beaudevin, 2017); or mostly in the public sector (in-house analyses in state-run sperm banks) as in the Chinese case studied by Wahlberg (2018). In parallel, new research endeavours involving not only DNA but also scientists from the global South have appeared, such as the Human Heredity and Health in Africa (H3Africa) initiative, which gathers members from a dozen of African countries (Fullwiley and Gibbon, 2018).

Against this backdrop, in 2011 the WHO replaced its medical genetics strategy with strong advocacy for 'genomics-based interventions for public health improvement in developing countries' (WHO, 2011), and in 2016 relabelled its Human Genetics Programme as Human Genomics in Global Health (WHO, 2018). In so doing the Organization explicitly turned to research activities in the field and presented genomics (especially in its 'stratified medicine' aspect) as a pathway to global health (Gibbon, chapter 8 in this volume).

The majority of financial investments in, and growing research and clinical uses of, genetics are still located in the global North. However, chronic disorders and risk-management strategies make up a massive part of global health initiatives in the South, and medical genetics and genomics tools are increasingly present in low- and middle-income countries. Investigating what global health does to medical genetics (and vice versa) means analysing the manifold local ways of doing genomic research, clinical and community genetics, i.e. the processes that lead – or not – to their integration into local priorities. The two chapters in this volume that address the globalization of genetics and genomics thus focus on the internationalization and coordination of research in genetics and genomics (Sturdy, chapter 7) and on the generalization of genetic testing services and prevention policies in Brazil (Gibbon, chapter 8). Following their analysis, the contemporary landscape of medical genetics on a global scale appears to be composed of various assemblages of screening and testing priorities, nosological and diagnostic discrepancies, clinical interactions, molecular tools, funding capacities and emerging markets. A distinctive trait – maybe a weakness – of globalized genetics is the heavy reliance of these assemblages on translational research and 'frontier' and promissory knowledge. The design of most genetic studies of human populations has thus recently shifted from families to populations, from rare to common diseases (Sturdy, chapter 7). What does this shift imply? What is the 'population' that is tackled by such studies? Further, the current definition of a population is closely related to the way(s) in which genetics, genomics and their clinical translations deal with diversity – and especially with one of its avatars, namely race. The scope and locations of population studies include more and more of the global South, thus changing the scientific status of DNA samples taken there. Such a situation, unsurprisingly, leads to the matter of race and its modes of existence in the clinic, where genetic testing for diagnosis purposes is performed, and articulated in a rather problematic manner with notions of community and choice (Gibbon, chapter 8).

The space occupied by genetics and genomics within contemporary global health is largely shaped by the concomitant dynamics of singularization and aggregation/quantification that penetrate the field of rare diseases, involving patients, scientists and physicians. These two rationales, which highlight alternatively the particularities of specific diseases or the shared ways in which various diseases affect myriads of people, compete when putting genetic and genomic medicine into the agenda of global health. As shown in the chapters by Gibbon and Sturdy, these rationales resonate in strikingly different ways according to the local context of their unfolding, most notably in relation to the local conceptions of race and to the ways in which health is considered (or not) as a fundamental right. In addition, the globalization of genetic and genomic medicine goes along with new understandings of communities and population, as well as a paradoxical 'renewed interest in finding molecular techniques for differentiating one population from another' (Sturdy, this volume). In the end, the design of investigations of the human genome in the search for disease genes require a definition of target groups that reinvigorate North–South divides (Sturdy, this volume). This colours genomic research with a shade of *déjà-vu* common to numerous global health endeavours.

The global health transition and the neoliberal turn

Neoliberalism is the ghost haunting the critical literature on global health (including our own). It is often understood as the domination of a market-centred political economy and ideology aiming at a minimal state and a drastic reduction of public services and social programmes. However, this definition proves to be too narrow and especially problematic in the area of health issues. Rather than the mere absence or the marginalization of the state, neoliberalism involves a *different* state from the Keynesian, developmentalist post-war one. The main function of the neoliberal state is to develop the institutions, the standards and the rules indispensable to creating and maintaining markets; hence, the centrality of intellectual property laws and the advocacy for public investment in the reproduction of human capital. Consider, for example, the sanitary turn of the World Bank in the 1990s, when the Bank started emphasizing health improvements as a path towards economic growth. Contrary to what observers have sometimes written, it cannot be reduced to privatization. The continuity with structural adjustment programmes is elsewhere. The Bank started to appeal for massive but 'cost-efficient' public investment in health programmes and infrastructure, omitting the biomedical model of high-tech hospitals benefiting the urban middle-class in favour of economically validated primary health care interventions (Gaudillière and Gasnier, 2020).

Approaching this turn therefore implies focusing on both the institutional reorganization and the tools involved in such optimization and prioritization of public investment in health. Examining the trajectory of the WHO, in chapter 9 Nitsan Chorev argues that the rise of the

World Bank as a dominant actor in global health challenged the WHO by establishing an 'external' logic of action that, in keeping with neoliberalism, prioritized cost-effectiveness in the choice and ranking of needs and paths of public interventions. This triggered an 'internal' strategic adaptation within the WHO. The main outcome of this alignment was to incorporate not only the discourse of health as a central determinant of economic growth but also the tools associated with performance (from the DALYs [disability-adjusted life years] calculus to the public-private partnerships). It also adapted them to the pursuit of WHO goals, thus providing continuity with the ways in which the selective primary health care policies of the 1970s and 1980s sought to tackle the problem of scarcity. In addition to this institutional shift and adaptation, one may argue that the broader managerial turn in governance was also central to global health; more central than the processes of privatization and/or austerity policies. The rise of the World Bank's language and tools accompanying the emergence of global health came with the new centrality and pervasive role of budget balancing and triage and performance, ideally based on cost-benefit assessment (Gaudillière and Gasnier, 2020).

Beyond the reconfiguration of governance and the enlarged palette of targets, 'cognitive' markers of the transition are equally important in characterizing a regime of global health in the making. In his epilogue to this volume Didier Fassin singles out two important candidates that previous chapters allude to but do not discuss up front. The first is pharmaceuticalization, with the centrality given to interventions focusing on drugs, their invention, commercialization, access and use. The second is the emphasis on risk management as the referent framework for handling unexpected epidemiological transitions, such as the prevalence of chronic pathologies affecting people in higher- and middle-income countries; and the simultaneous (re)-emergence and 'chronicization' of diseases like malaria, tuberculosis and AIDS, creating the unprecedented types and numbers of patients affected with multiple pathologies. Reflecting on these as well as other possible traits accounting for the specificity of global health, Fassin suggests that the field of global health operates along multiple lines of tensions between the spatial and the ideological, the moral and the economic, the trends toward compassion and predation, all of which illustrate the violence and the critical potential of global health.

The past and the future of global health

Global health as it is practised and debated often appears short sighted, more concerned with challenges and how they are to be met rather than with how they were made and what their future may look like. In a popular critical piece Anne-Emanuelle Birn (2005) has dissected the Gates Foundation's 'grandest challenge' of 2003. As she convincingly argues, it actively neglects a large part of what are challenges for global health, instead insisting on a technological solution for current problems and ignoring that these problems have a history that suggests that social policy approaches are equally promising. Critical analyses of global health are in need of expanded horizons. The present volume has taken up that challenge. Rather than depending on classical historiography, we historicize the turning point around 1990. History resides on both sides of this divide. As the emblematic case of TB control and DOTS shows, the turn took place between the mid-1980s and the late 1990s. However, the arrival of global health with efficiency-focused metrics and donor-driven interventions was at the same time a revival of vertical, technology-driven approaches pushed back during the period of the WHO's primary health care policy. The internal dynamics of global health became even more visible and encompassing when global TB control turned to drug resistance and its control after 2005.

This book presents global health not simply as an agenda but, rather, as a regime, with a beginning, that will arguably be replaced at some point in time by another regime. The anthropological contributions in the volume provide impressive illustrations of the dynamics at work here. Asian medicines, for instance, can be approached through their role in the making of global health, yet the chapters in this book show them to have a potential far beyond that. They are better understood within a larger geopolitics of the twenty-first century, characterized by South–South relations dominated by a strong presence of South-East Asian actors. Within this perspective, analyses of global health from 1990 to 2010 become a search-light pointing towards a twenty-first-century global political order.

The four domains explored in this book not only reveal decisive differences regarding the paths through which localization and generalization have been worked out. Their comparison also highlights contrasted modes of insertion within global health as a field. TB control is, in this respect, the most integrated, with large investments by big (international) players and nation-states, the design of a standardized intervention package and a clearly vertical organization of programmes. In contrast, the globalization of Asian medicines is marginally achieved through global health institutions. It operates through processes of circulation (of goods, practitioners and patients), with their limitations and specific regulations, rather than through programmes and public investments. Medical genetics and mental health reveal intermediary configurations that juxtapose significant discursive visibility and the absence of large investments of resources in the field. Consequently, programmes, when they exist, are often experimental, locally or nationally designed, and build on local epidemiology and epistemic choices. Articulating anthropological and historical approaches thus appears essential to understanding why such differences emerged and how they impact on the globalization of health.

More generally, the exchanges between the observations and methods of anthropology and history that this volume advocates are crucial for keeping a critical eye on these processes. Studying a dynamic phenomenon like global health requires close attention both to its actual state of being and to the paths of its development over time. This book shows how the history of twentieth century genetics seems likely to be rewritten from the perspective of the rise of the contemporary genetic services industry, and the discourse of human rights in mental health assumes the revolutionizing of the means of treating people with mental illnesses situated in time and place. This does not make anthropologists out of historians, or vice versa. Rather, the book illustrates how the skilful combination of insights from both of these disciplines provides for a richer and more critical approach to global health and to the regimes of practice it that fosters, with their impact, contradictions and limitations.

References

Adams, V. (2016) 'Metrics of the global sovereign: numbers and stories in global health', in V. Adams (ed.), *Metrics: What Count in Global Health*. Durham: Duke University Press, 19–54.

Alter, J. S. (ed.) (2005) *Asian Medicine and Globalization*. Philadelphia: University of Pennsylvania Press.
Amrith, S. (2006) *Decolonizing International Health: India and Southeast Asia, 1930–65*. Basingstoke: Palgrave Macmillan.
Banerjee, M. (2009) *Power, Knowledge, Medicine: Ayurvedic Pharmaceuticals at Home and in the World*. New Delhi: Orient Black Swan Pvt Ltd.
Beaudevin, C. (2017) 'Arabian medical genetics: of rare disorders and decreasing oil rent', in *Medizinethnologie. Körper, Gesundheit und Heilung in einer globalisierten Welt*, http://www.medizinethnologie.net/arabian-medical-genetics.
Behrouzan, O. (2016) *Prozak Diaries: Psychiatry and Generational Memory in Iran*. Stanford: Stanford University Press.
Bhattacharya, S. (2006) *Expunging Variola: The Control and Eradication of Smallpox in India, 1947–1977*. New Delhi and London: Orient Longman India and Sangam Books.
Birn, A.-E. (2005) 'Gates's grandest challenge: transcending technology as public health ideology', *The Lancet* 366 (9484), 514–519.
Birn, A.-E. (2009) 'The stages of international (global) health: histories of success or successes of history?', *Global Public Health* 4 (1), 50–68.
Bode, M. (2008) *Taking Traditional Knowledge to the Market. The Modern Image of the Ayurvedic and Unani Industry 1980–2000*. Hyderabad: Orient Longman.
Brimnes, N. (2016) *Languished Hopes. Tuberculosis, the State and International Assistance in Twentieth Century India*. Hyderabad: Orient Black Swan.
Brown, H., Kelly, A. H. (2014) 'Material proximities and hotspots: toward an anthropology of viral hemorrhagic fevers', *Medical Anthropology Quarterly* 28 (2), 280–303.
Brown, T., Cueto, M., Fee, E. (2006) 'The World Health Organization and the transition from "international" to "global" public health', *American Journal of Public Health* 96 (1), 62–72.
Carothers, J. C. (1953) *The African Mind in Health and Disease. A Study in Ethnopsychiatry*. Geneva: WHO.
Cassier, M., Correa, M. (2003) 'Patents, innovation and public health: Brazilian public-sector laboratories' experience in copying AIDS drugs', in J-P. Moatti et al. (eds), *Economics of AIDS and Access to HIV/AIDS Care in Developing Countries. Issues and Challenge*. Paris: Editions ANRS, 89–107.
Chorev, N. (2012) *The World Health Organization between North and South*. Ithaca: Cornell University Press.
Coderey, C., Pordié, L. (2019) *Circulation and Governance of Asian Medicine*. London/New York: Routledge.

Condrau, F., Worboys, M. (2010) *Tuberculosis Then and Now/ Perspectives on the History of an Infectious Disease*. Montreal: McGill-Queen's University Press.

Craig, S., Adams, V. (2008) 'Global pharma in the land of snows. Tibetan medicines, SARS, and identity politics across nations', *Asian Medicine* 4 (1), 1–28.

Cueto, M. (2007) *Cold War, Deadly Fevers: Malaria Eradication in Mexico, 1955–1975*. Baltimore: Johns Hopkins University Press.

Cueto, M., Brown. T., Fee, E. (2019) *The World Health Organization: A History*. Cambridge: Cambridge University Press.

de Chadarevian, S. (2015) 'Human population studies and the World Health Organisation', *Dynamis* 35 (2), 359–388.

Desjarlais, R. (1995) *World Mental Health: Problems and Priorities in Low-income Countries*. New York: Oxford University Press.

Droney, D. (2014) 'Ironies of laboratory work during Ghana's second age of optimism', *Cultural Anthropology* 29 (2), 363–384.

Dumit, J. (2012) *Drugs for Life: How Pharmaceutical Companies Define Our Health*. Durham, NC: Duke University Press.

Ernst, W. (2013) *Colonialism and Transnational Psychiatry: The Development of an Indian Hospital in British India, 1925–1940*. New York: Anthem Press.

Farmer, P., Sen, A. (2004) *Pathologies of Power: Health, Human Right and the New War on the Poor*. Berkeley: University of California Press.

Fassin, D., Rechtman, R. (2009) *The Empire of Trauma. An Inquiry in the Condition of Victimhood*. Princeton, NJ: Princeton University Press.

Fullwiley, D., Gibbon, S. (2018) 'Genomics in emerging and developing economies', in S. Gibbon, B. Prainsack, S. Hilgartner, and J. Lamoreaux (eds), *Handbook of Genomics, Health and Society*. London, New York: Routledge, 228–237.

Gaudillière, J-P., Hess, V. (eds) (2013) *Ways of Regulating Drugs in the 19th and 20th Centuries*. Basingstoke and New York: Palgrave Macmillan.

Gaudillière, J-P., Thoms, U. (eds) (2015) *The Development of Scientific Marketing in the Twentieth Century*. New York: Pickering & Chatto.

Gaudillière, J-P., Gasnier, C. (2020) 'From Washington DC to Washington state: the global burden of diseases data basis and the political economy of global health', in S. Leonelli and N. Tempini (eds), *Data Journeys in the Sciences*. New York: Springer, 321–339.

Gaudillière, J-P., Beaudevin, C., Lang, C., McDowell, A. (forthcoming) *The Health of Others: Global Health, Knowledge, Politics*.

Geissler, P. W. (ed.) (2015) *Para-States and Medical Science: Making African Global Health*. Critical Global Health. Durham, NC: Duke University Press.

Geissler, P. W., Lachenal, G., Manton, J., Tousignant N. (eds) (2016) *Traces of the Future. An Archaeology of Medical Science in Africa*. Chicago: Chicago University Press.
Gibbon, S. (2013) 'Ancestry, Temporality, and Potentiality. Engaging Cancer Genetics in Southern Brazil', *Current Anthropology* 54 (7), 107–117.
Gibbon, S., Waleska, A. (2018) 'Inclusion and exclusion in the globalisation of genomics; the case of rare genetic disease in Brazil', *Anthropology & Medicine* 25 (1), 11–29.
Graboyes, M. (2015) *The Experiment Must Continue: Medical Research and Ethics in East Africa, 1940–2014*. Athens: Ohio University Press.
Gradmann, C. (2019) 'Treatment on trial: Tanzania's National Tuberculosis Programme, the International Union against Tuberculosis and Lung Disease, and the Road to Dots, 1977–1991', *Journal of the History of Medicine and Allied Sciences* 74, 316–343.
Greene, J. A. (2007) *Prescribing by Numbers: Drugs and the Definition of Disease*. Baltimore: Johns Hopkins University Press.
Greene, J. A. (2014) *Generic. The Unbranding of Modern Medicine*. Baltimore: Johns Hopkins University Press.
Harper, I. (2010) 'Extreme conditions, extreme measures: compliance, drug resistance and the control of tuberculosis', *Anthropology & Medicine* 17, 201–214.
Horwitz, A., Wakefield, J. C. (2007) *The Loss of Sadness: How Psychiatry Transformed Normal Sorrow into Depressive Disorder*. New York: Oxford University Press.
Howard-Jones, N. (1981) *The Pan-American Health Organization: Origins and Evolution*. Geneva: World Health Organization.
Hunt, N. R. (2015) *A Nervous State: Violence, Remedies, and Reverie in Colonial Congo*. Durham, NC: Duke University Press.
Hyman, S. E. (2010) 'The diagnosis of mental disorders: the problem of reification', *Annual Review of Clinical Anthropology* 6, 155–179.
Keller, R. C. (2008) *Colonial Madness: Psychiatry in French North Africa*. Chicago: University of Chicago Press.
Kim, J. Y., Shakow, A., Mate, K., Vanderwaker, C., Gupta, R., Farmer, P. (2005) 'Limited good and limited vision: multidrug resistant tuberculosis and global health policy', *Social Science & Medicine* 61, 847–859.
Kleinman, A. (2012) 'Culture, bereavement and psychiatry', *The Lancet* 379 (9816), 608–609.
Kohrt, B. A., Mendenhall, E. (2016) *Global Mental Health: Anthropological Perspectives*. London: Routledge.
Lachenal, G. (2014) *Le medicament qui devait sauver l'Afrique. Un scandale pharmaceutique aux colonies*. Paris: La Découverte.

Lang, C., Jansen, E. (2013) 'Appropriating depression: biomedicalizing ayurvedic psychiatry in Kerala, India', *Medical Anthropology* 32 (1), 25–45.
Langwick, S. A. (2015) 'Partial publics: the political promise of traditional medicine in Africa', *Current Anthropology* 56 (4), 493–514.
Lee, K. (2009) *The World Health Organization*. London: Routledge.
Lee, S. (1997) 'WHO and the developing world: the contest for ideology', in A. Cunningham and B. Andrews (eds), *Western Medicine as Contested Knowledge* (pp. 24–45). Manchester: Manchester University Press.
Lindee, S. (2014) 'Scaling up: human genetics as a Cold War network', *Studies in History and Philosophy of Biological and Biomedical Sciences* 47, 185–190.
Litsios, S. (1997) 'Malaria control, rural development and the postwar reordering of international organizations', *Medical Anthropology* 14, 255–278.
Livingston, J. (2012) *Improvising Medicine: An African Oncology Ward in an Emerging Cancer Epidemics*. Durham, NC: Duke University Press.
Lock, M., Nguyen, V. K. (2018) *An Anthropology of Biomedicine*. New York: Wiley & Sons.
Lovell, A. (2014) 'The World Health Organization and the contested beginnings of psychiatric epidemiology as an international discipline: one rope, many strands', *International Journal of Epidemiology* 43 (suppl 1), i6–i18.
McMillen, C. (2015) *Discovering Tuberculosis. A Global History, 1900 to the Present*. New Haven: Yale University Press.
Modell, B., Kuliev, A. (1998) 'The history of community genetics: the contribution of the haemoglobin disorders', *Community Genetics* 1, 3–11.
Muraskin, W. (2005) *Crusade to Immunize the World's Children: The Origin of the Bill and Melinda Gates Children's Vaccine Programme and the Birth of the Global Alliance for Vaccines and Immunization*. Los Angeles: Global BioBusiness Book.
Murray, C., Lopez, A. D. (1996) *Global Burden of Disease*. Cambridge, MA: Harvard University Press.
Packard, R. (1989) *White Plague, Black Labor. Tuberculosis and the Political Economy of Health and Disease in South Africa*. Berkeley: University of California Press.
Packard, R. (2016) *A History of Global Health. Interventions into the Lives of Other Peoples*. Baltimore: Johns Hopkins University Press.
Page, B., Valone, D. (eds) (2007) *Philanthropic Foundations and the Globalization of Scientific Medicine and Public Health*. Lanham, MD: University Press of America.
Petryna, A. (2009) *When Experiments Travel: Clinical Trials and the Global Search for Human Subject*. Princeton, NJ: Princeton University Press.

Petryna, A. et al. (2006) *Global Pharmaceuticals: Ethics, Markets, Practices*. Durham, NC: Duke University Press.

Pordié, L. (ed.) (2011) 'Savoirs thérapeutiques asiatiques et mondialisation', *Revue d'Anthropologie des Connaissances* 5 (1), 3–12. DOI: 10.3917/rac.012.0003.

Pordié, L. (2014) 'Pervious drugs. Making the pharmaceutical object in techno-ayurveda', *Asian Medicine* 9 (1–2), 49–76.

Pordié, L., Gaudillière, J-P. (2014) 'The reformulation regime in drug discovery. Revisiting polyherbals and property rights in the Ayurvedic industry', *EASTS* 8, 57–79.

Rao, M. (ed.) (1999) *Disinvesting in Health: The World Bank's Prescriptions for Health*, Thousand Oaks, CA: Sage Publications.

Ruault, L., Beaudevin, C., Gaudillière, J-P., Geise, M. (forthcoming) 'What globalizing means – community genetics, 1971–2018'.

Siddiqi, J. (1995) *World Health and World Politics: The World Health Organization and the UN System*. London: Hurst.

Staples, A. (2006) *The Birth of Development: How the World Bank, Food and Agriculture Organization, and World Health Organization Have Changed the World 1945–1965*. Kent, OH: Kent State University Press.

Tousignant, N. (2012) 'Trypanosomes, toxicity and resistance: the politics of mass therapy in French colonial Africa', *Social History of Medicine* 25 (3), 625–643.

Van Os, J. et al. (2009) 'A systematic review and meta-analysis of the psychosis continuum: evidence for a psychosis proneness-persistence-impairment model of psychotic disorder', *Psychological Medicine* 39 (2), 179–195.

Wahlberg, A. (2018) *Good Quality. The Routinization of Sperm Banking in China*. Berkeley: University of California Press.

Webb, J. (2008) *Humanity's Burden: A Global History of Malaria*. Cambridge: Cambridge University Press.

Weisz, G., Cambrosio, A., Cointet, J-P. (2017) 'Mapping global health: a network analysis of a heterogeneous publication domain', *Biosocieties* 12 (4), 520–542.

White, R. G. et al. (2017) *The Palgrave Handbook of Sociocultural Perspectives on Global Mental Health*. New York: Springer.

WHO (1981) *Health for All by the Year 2000: The Contribution of Human Genetics. Report of the Task Group on Genetics Programme*. Geneva: WHO.

WHO (2011) *Grand Challenges in Genomics for Public Health in Developing Countries. Top 10 Policy and Research Priorities to Harness Genomics for the Greatest Public Health Problems*. Geneva: WHO.

WHO (2018) *Human Genomics in Global Health*, www.who.int/genomics/en/ (accessed 12 January 2018).

World Bank (1993) *World Development Report 1993: Investing in Health*. New York: World Bank. https://openknowledge.worldbank.org/handle/10986/5976 (accessed 25 February 2020).

Wu, H. (2015) 'World citizenship and the emergence of the social psychiatry project of the WHO, 1948–1965', *History of Psychiatry* 26 (2), 166–181.

Young, A. (1997) *The Harmony of Illusions: Inventing Post-Traumatic Stress Disorder*. Princeton, NJ: Princeton University Press.

Zhan, M. (2009) *Other-Worldly: Making Chinese Medicine through Transnational Frames*. Durham, NC: Duke University Press.

2
Standardization and localization in tuberculosis control

Nora Engel

Introduction

Standardized drug-delivery programmes, such as tuberculosis (TB) control programmes, are often promoted as universal solutions that allow using the same training modules, delivery strategies, technologies and logistics across very different contexts. They promise (cost-) efficiency, and to reach large populations quickly, while generating comparable global data through the same reporting and recording guidelines and standards. Yet, when controlling TB and implementing such seemingly universal solutions across different settings, contexts and social worlds of actors, there is a central tension between standardization and localization; between programmatic considerations and responding to individual care needs, including particular TB strains, comorbidities, personal pharmaceutical histories or socio-economic circumstances. Making this tension work acquires particular urgency in the case of TB, where failing treatment can exacerbate amplification and transmission of drug resistance. What is more, the rise of MDR-TB (multi-drug resistant tuberculosis) has intensified the basic tension between responding to individual care needs and standardizing treatment. In India the tension between standardization and localization has been described as one of the major challenges for MDR-TB treatment (Engel, 2015). Diagnosis, treatment, follow-up test schedules, reporting and recording activities are longer and more extensive and complicated than in routine TB treatment. Drug-resistance patterns vary from patient to patient and across time, and the risk of medical complications is high. Patients often need more support. They likely have spent years with unsuccessful TB treatment, are frustrated, impoverished and exhausted. The treatment is more toxic, longer, costlier and more difficult to bear than routine TB treatment, with only a 60% chance of cure. Yet adapting treatment regimens individually requires advanced laboratory diagnostics, complicated follow-up investigations, more resources, counsellors and other forms of social and financial support. All of which are often impossible to provide in public health contexts. National TB programmes thus apply standardized drug regimens and drug-delivery processes to make the treatment sustainable and replicable across localities, to ensure that the risk of transmission of infectious strains is limited and the potential amplification of drug-resistance is avoided. These standards are constrained by local and health-system capacities.

This chapter examines the tension between standardization and localization in efforts to control TB through the DOTS strategy. It uses anthropological and sociological literature that has (often critically) discussed the DOTS strategy and examples from past empirical fieldwork in 2008 and 2009 at an MDR-TB treatment site in India.

Standardized protocols, guidelines, artefacts, curricula and policies are widely used to orchestrate and control health care delivery and are believed to ensure quality, reliability and comparability in health outcomes as long as they are being implemented 'correctly'. Implementation research in health sciences has aimed at closing the potential gap between such standards and real-life practices (Bhattacharyya, Reeves and Zwarenstein, 2009). Science and Technology Studies scholars showed that standardization requires continuous work and renegotiation and is precisely not a matter of the straightforward implementation of a standard (Bowker and Star, 1999; Lampland and Star, 2009; Timmermans and Epstein, 2010; Zeiss, 2004). During the development of standardized guidelines, protocols or policies, universal standards and local practices continuously interact (Timmermans and Berg, 2003). This means that universal standards do not always work in every locality and might mean different things (Anderson, 2006; Lampland and Star, 2009; Lock and Nguyen, 2010; Petryna, 2009). In order to function in specific situations, standards have to become universalised locals (Timmermans and Berg, 1997), actors need to arrive at forms of situated standardization (Zuiderent-Jerak, 2007a), for instance in a workflow of reflexive standardization (Timmermans, 2015). Universals are thus locally contingent, complex and negotiated constructs (Timmermans and Epstein, 2010). Viewed in this way, standardization in TB control is ongoing, localized, emerging, negotiated and based on prior routines and relations. The interest is then to understand how actors enact standards in practices, rather than to suggest a particular balance of local adaptation and standardization (Engel and Zeiss, 2014). Such an approach allows studying how patients and health care providers negotiate what for them is social about TB, instead of taking social determinants as taken for granted in advance (Koch, 2016). In what follows and after a brief background on DOTS, the existing critique on DOTS is reviewed with regard to the relationship between standardization and localization and discussed with empirical results from earlier fieldwork at an MDR-TB treatment site in India.

DOTS and DOTS Plus in India

The DOTS strategy (directly observed treatment, short course) consists of five elements: government commitment, case detection by sputum microscopy, standardized treatment regimens of six to eight months with direct observation (DOT) for at least the initial two months, regular supply of anti-TB drugs and a standardized recording and reporting system (WHO, 2002). DOTS is centred on a biomedical model of TB, reducing transmission of TB by treating patients with anti-TB drugs. The disease is viewed as a managerial problem that can be solved with drugs. Consequently, the main problem addressed by the strategy is non-adherence to those drugs and not, for instance, prevention of TB.

In a coordinated approach between the World Bank offering soft loans conditional on implementing DOTS in endemic countries, bilateral agencies providing supplementary support and the WHO with its technical guidance, the DOTS strategy was being implemented globally throughout the 1990s. Implementation is organized in vertical disease-control programmes and, to varying degrees, integrated into the general health services. According to the WHO, the DOTS strategy saved an estimated 49 million lives between 2000 and 2015 (http://www.who.int/tb/en/). It has been labelled as 'one of the most widely-implemented and longest-running global health interventions in history' (Obermeyer, Abbott-Klafter and Murray, 2008).

In India, the Revised National Tuberculosis Control Programme (RNTCP) with DOTS at its core was implemented from 1997. The RNTCP replaced the former National TB Programme, which a programmatic review in 1992 attested to be suffering from managerial weaknesses, inadequate funding, over-reliance on X-ray for diagnosis, frequent interrupted supplies of drugs and low rates of treatment completion (Agarwal, Vijay, Kumar and Chauhan, 2005; Nagpaul, 1999; Narayan, 1998). The coordinated approach between the World Bank, WHO and bilateral agencies in implementing DOTS left little policy space for alternative voices or concerns about DOTS in the TB community, such as TB patients, practitioners and community TB workers. What is more, the TB community at that time was unorganized, demotivated, underfunded and under-resourced and the private health care sector had grown expansively and remains largely unregulated (Walt, 1999).

The RNTCP is a vertical disease-control programme with separate administrative, governance, funding and reporting structures, yet is integrated into the general health services from sub-district level onwards. It is a passive case-finding programme, meaning that patients need to present to the RNTCP to be diagnosed. A sputum smear microscopy test is performed at one of the district microscopy centres and patients are assigned to one of the highly standardized treatment categories. Treatment is initiated by the medical officer in the respective TB unit. The patient is referred to a DOTS provider in his/her vicinity who stores the box containing the full treatment course, reports adherence to treatment and follows up patients who have not been taking their drugs. During the intensive phase of at least two months, the patient has to take the drugs every alternate day under the supervision of the DOTS provider, who ticks off the boxes on the TB treatment card for each visit. In the continuation phase the patient is supervised only during the first dose of each week when collecting the weekly tablet strips from the DOTS provider and during random visits by health workers. A patient is considered cured when the result of the sputum test changes from positive to negative bacilli load in the last month of treatment and on at least one previous occasion (Central TB Division, 2005). The targets that should be reached are: to cure 90% of all newly detected pulmonary TB cases and 85% for re-treatment cases, and to achieve a 90% notification rate for all cases (Central TB Division, 2016).

Many have judged the RNTCP as a success story, particularly because of its internationally unprecedented rapid expansion across the country and the rigour that it brought to the health system. Yet there are also considerable critical voices with regard to the quality of care provided and how the programme has handled the challenges related to drug resistance, as will become clear below (Chakraborty, 2003; Engel, 2013; Udwadia and Pinto, 2007). Furthermore, the RNTCP does not extend into the vast private sector. The quality of TB care in India has been shown to be suboptimal in numerous studies, especially in the private sector (Satyanarayana et al., 2015). The majority of private providers are not able to prescribe a correct TB treatment and have not been contacted by the public TB programme. In a now classic study in a poor neighbourhood in Mumbai, 100 private providers reported prescribing eighty different regimens, most of them inappropriate and expensive (Uplekar and Rangan, 1993). In a follow-up study in the same area two decades later nothing much seemed to have changed: 106 providers reported prescribing sixty-three different regimens for their TB patients (Udwadia, Pinto and Uplekar, 2010). And there is a big gap between what providers claim they do when they suspect TB, or their knowledge about TB treatment, and what they actually do to diagnose and treat TB patients (J. Das et al., 2015). Many private providers treat empirically, based on symptoms, at least initially. Non-specialist providers commonly use medications as diagnostic tools, meaning that only when several of their broad-spectrum regimens are failing will they suspect TB (McDowell and Pai, 2016).

What is more, DOTS assumes that public health systems are strong enough to manage such a complex intervention (Banerji, 1998; Seeberg, 2014). Yet in some places problems with infrastructure, maintenance of equipment, retention of staff, vacancies and irregular staff presence and limited opening hours of clinics jeopardise the implementation of DOTS. As Jens Seeberg highlights, the rapid expansion across the country in combination with a weak health system came at the cost of considerably increasing the number of defaulters and those unable to complete the treatment – uncured patients at high risk of developing MDR-TB (Seeberg, 2014) (see below, DOTS is causing MDR-TB).

Initially DOTS did not take into account MDR-TB. It was only in 1999 that the WHO started to develop an approach, and in 2006 global DOTS Plus guidelines for diagnosis and treatment of MDR-TB were published. Pilot sites for treating MDR-TB had been set up across different countries with large numbers of TB patients. In India, DOTS Plus was piloted from 2007 and nationally adapted guidelines were published in 2010. According to these guidelines, MDR-TB treatment takes twenty-four to twenty-seven months, as opposed to six to eight months for routine TB treatment. During the intensive phase of six months, patients need to visit their DOTS provider daily to receive an injection of medication and swallow ten to thirteen different drugs (drugs only on Sundays, no injection) under direct observation. The subsequent continuation phase involves only tablets and the patient needs to take only the first dose of each week under supervision (Central TB Division, 2010). Today MDR-TB treatment is part of general TB treatment. The challenges of implementing DOTS within the given constraints of the health system and adhering to treatment are intensified for MDR-TB.

Debates around DOTS

Medicalization of the problem does not do justice to socio-cultural contexts and individual needs

One of the main points of critique about DOTS is that the DOTS strategy has a strong focus on case management and generally lacks attention to social factors such as poverty (Enarson and Billo, 2007). The RNTCP in India, much like its predecessor the national TB programme, continued with a dominant biomedical frame wherein techno-managerial interventions are emphasized (Narayan, 1998). This strong medicalization of the problem of TB has direct consequences for the control strategies that focus, for instance, on patient education and supervision as measures to overcome default, because default is understood as a fault of patients (Narayan, 1999). Sociological literature has long criticized the notion of patients' compliance with medication for placing the main responsibility for treatment failure on patients, leading to victim-blaming (Ogden, 1999; Williams, 2001), for being judgemental (Lerner, 1997) and for representing a form of medical control that reduces patients to passive recipients of biomedical instructions and ignores patients' perspectives (Conrad, 1992; Mykhalovskiy, McCoy and Bresalier, 2004). The medical sociology and anthropology literature has emphasized how structural factors such as poverty, economic inequality, political violence, social stratification and marginality rather than individual, rational decision making by patients determine care-seeking behaviour and adherence to treatment or advice (V. Das and Das, 2006; Farmer, 1997, 2003). Structural barriers were more important than cultural differences (often located in patients) in the production of non-adherence to TB treatment in Haiti (Farmer, 1997), Bolivia (Greene, 2004) and Nepal (Harper, 2005a). Seeking care and adhering to treatment is determined by social and economic factors and the physical side-effects of drugs (Noyes and Popay, 2007). Common themes that deter adhering to DOTS include the indirect or hidden costs of adhering to treatment, relationships between providers and patients, patients' ability to make sense of the intervention in multiple frames of reference, importance of gender (Noyes and Popay, 2007), other forms of discrimination (Greene, 2004), stigma (Isaakidis et al., 2013) and severe side-effects, especially for adhering to MDR-TB treatment (Deshmukh et al., 2015; Isaakidis et al., 2013). Harper's ethnographic work in Nepal also shows how DOTS implementation is complicated by stigma, difficulties in accessing DOTS centres, caste relationships between providers and patients and strong social hierarchies within the health system that do not allow for the suggestion of more flexibility in implementing DOTS to superiors in the programme (Harper, 2005a). The strong medicalization thus ignores the health system status and context of patients. If, by contrast, default were understood as poor management or as a result of systemic failures of the health service, then the solution would entail increased funding, the improvement of infrastructural functioning and capacity building in public health services (Narayan, 1999).

Responding to this lethal combination of structural violence, sociocultural factors and harsh side-effects requires tremendous effort, and work by both patients and providers. Harper suggests that for routine TB in Nepal providers can generally make adherence work if conditions and supervision are supportive and existing social hierarchies are taken into account:

> Given the right conditions and supervisory support, most of the staff would work out appropriate strategies for dealing with the vexed

question of adherence to treatment. This requires a different relationship, however, with the staff, and an understanding of how the rigid requirements of a research agenda linked to the health service can feed counterproductively (from the perspective of patient support) into already existing social hierarchies. (Harper, 2005a: 63)

Yet the additional challenges of MDR-TB complicate those responses further. A team of researchers at a Médecins sans Frontières clinic in Mumbai, India that provides treatment for MDR-TB patients co-infected with HIV warn that the resources required to ensure patients adhere to current long-term regimens are very demanding. And even if resources are available and free treatment is offered, with services going far beyond those currently offered in public clinics, patients find it extremely difficult to adhere due to the harsh side-effects and the heavy social and financial burdens of long-term treatment and illness with stigmatized diseases (Isaakidis et al., 2013). Because the problem of TB is highly medicalized, the standardization of TB control in DOTS does not do justice to socio-cultural contexts and individual care needs and to the tremendous efforts that it takes to respond to structural factors and individual needs.

DOTS can cause MDR-TB: narrow epidemiological categories and target orientation

The standardization necessary to generate comparable data on the epidemiology of TB is marginalizing some patients from treatment. The DOTS strategy is criticized for its focus on cutting transmission by treating patients who suffer from infectious pulmonary TB (diagnosis is focused on sputum positive). Patients who are non-infectious to others receive less attention and their diagnosis and treatment is of lower priority (such as sputum negative or extra-pulmonary TB) (Narayan, 1999). Ian Harper showed that the biomedical categories of DOTS, which define different TB patients as newly diagnosed, retreatment, relapse and failure cases, do not always match the treatment and pharmaceutical history of patients in Nepal, especially in the absence of on-the-spot testing for extra-pulmonary or drug-resistant forms of TB. By generating non-eligible TB patients and turning them away the programme might be creating MDR-TB and, worse, not knowingly, because those patients who are not allowed into the programme are not being counted or diagnosed for MDR-TB. They will ultimately not show up in national databases (Harper, 2005a). Narrow epidemiological disease categories that deny access to treatment to those patients who fall outside these categories are a form of structural violence (Farmer, 1998, 2003). The focus on reducing transmission represents a technical fix that does not attempt to address in a comprehensive way the reasons why TB is a problem, and will ultimately fail in combination with a weak health system (Banerji, 1998). Taking this point further, Seeberg argues that making MDR-TB treatment available through DOTS Plus without addressing the syndemic dynamics of the disease (its social, historical and political context, its close relation to social inequality, comorbidity, malnutrition, poor living conditions and poverty) and the practices of the unregulated Indian private sector (where most TB patients seek care first and are often diagnosed too late and wrongly treated) amount to the medicalization of poverty, which is ultimately creating further drug resistance (Seeberg, 2014).

The standardization of TB control not only marginalizes some patients from treatment, it also allows for rapid expansion of treatment access, but at the cost of quality because of weak health system services (see above). Seeberg shows powerfully how the standardized approach and reliance on targets lead to fudging numbers, trickle down and put pressure on the professional hierarchy (Seeberg, 2014). District TB officers whose quarterly numbers of detection and cure rates do not meet targets are reprimanded by their superiors at state level, who have to answer to central-level officers and thus are likely to hide poor performance. At sub-district level senior treatment supervisors visit, supervise and counsel defaulting patients and the DOTS providers. Yet this supervision often equals reprimanding, scolding and blaming – at times publicly using social dynamics of class, stigma and gender. This strains already fragile relationships between DOTS providers and patients, so much so that DOTS providers ultimately blame patients for not adhering to treatment. It reinforces care seeking in the private sector, where treatment is costly, often of poor quality or inadequate, but shorter, unsupervised and confidential (Seeberg, 2014). However, technical fixes and target orientation are in line with international targets, funding requirements by large-scale donors and the general characteristics of vertical disease-control programmes. Questioning the success in creating access through such standards is difficult, even if they might be contributing to the emergence of MDR-TB (Seeberg,

2014). These concerns point to the risk that standardization of TB control in DOTS, in combination with a weak health system, is causing defaulters, marginalization and poor quality of care, and ultimately is generating MDR-TB.

Direct observation is paternalistic

The majority of the debate on DOTS has been targeted at the direct observation element. The benefits of directly observed therapy (DOT) versus self-administered therapy have been debated without clear outcome (Volmink and Garner, 2007; Zwarenstein, Schoeman, Vundule, Lombard and Tatley, 1998). DOTS is often characterized as a highly complex and paternalistic public health intervention, where the patient is seen as a passive recipient of care who cannot be trusted to adhere to treatment correctly and thus has to be observed (Ogden, 1999; Seeberg, 2014). DOT has been criticized for being an unethical and authoritative disease-control strategy (Narayan, 1998, 1999; Ogden, 2000; Pronyk and Porter, 1999) and for assuming that patients need to be controlled in order to avoid treatment failure and protect the drugs from losing their power (Craig, 2007; Harper, 2005b). In the RNTCP the patient is directly observed during the intensive phase of the treatment in the first two months for routine TB and during the first six months for MDR-TB treatment. Critics argue that the direct observation stops at a phase in the treatment where the patient starts feeling better symptomatically and is thus more likely to default (Udwadia and Pinto, 2007). DOT can in some cases deter adherence (Garner and Volmink, 2003). Despite the fact that DOT was promoted to overcome non-adherence, it ignores the obstacles that mainly the poor face when accessing health services (such as life circumstances and social class barriers) (Narayan, 1998). What is more, the targets of a rigid DOT programme may compete with the needs of patients when staff do not register those diagnosed patients who they think may not adhere (Bhargava, Pinto and Pai, 2011). Thus, DOT needs to be more flexible and support strategies need to be more diverse (Bhargava, Pinto and Pai, 2011; Garner and Volmink, 2003).

Since the late 1990s the WHO has weakened its strong focus on DOT and acknowledged that implementation of DOT without additional supportive measures is not successful (Maher, Gupta, Uplekar, Dye and Raviglione, 2000; Raviglione and Uplekar, 2006). Several studies have suggested that DOT is not implemented the same way in every context (Macq, Theobald, Dick and Dembele, 2003; Noyes and Popay, 2007). A systematic review of qualitative research on DOT showed that the variants of DOT differ in important ways in how direct observation is practised – for instance, who it is that is being observed, where the observation takes place and how often it occurs. These elements seem to determine the effect of DOT types on cure rates (Noyes and Popay, 2007). The expanded DOTS strategy of the Global TB Programme explicitly calls for making DOT more acceptable to patients (WHO, 2002). This represents an important discursive shift in global TB control (Harper, 2010): although senior staff at the WHO claimed that DOTS has always been more than direct observation, the branding as DOTS puts observation of patients centre stage in the acronym itself (Ogden, Walt and Lush, 2003). This shifted with the expanded StopTB strategy, where patient support and human rights language are part of the discourse as well (Harper, 2010).

Yet global TB control is grappling with a central tension and trade-off between patient-centred forms of TB care and how to prevent the emergence of resistance. According to Harper, the threat of drug resistance may jeopardize the nascent moves towards more patient-centredness in TB control, because of the urge to control and possibly sanction or detain patients so as to ensure adherence to a treatment that is increasingly difficult for patients to bear and for underfunded public health systems to provide, monitor and support (Harper, 2010). A similar tension has been noted for the Indian TB community (Engel, 2015). While the Indian RNTCP have announced the aim to put patients at the centre of their efforts, to make them 'very important persons', according to Bhargava and colleagues, these goals still need to be realized (Bhargava et al., 2011). In the 2016 guidelines the RNTCP has loosened the grip on direct observation in accordance with global policy shifts and now recommends to apply the principle of direct observation judiciously as and when the situation of the patient permits, and emphasizes a patient-centric model of care (Central TB Division, 2016). It remains to be seen how these flexibilities will be enacted in practice.

Overall, the discussion of the critique of the globally standardized treatment approach DOTS shows that standardization is often viewed as opposing, denying or limiting local adaptation to socio-cultural contexts and patients' needs. And, worse, that without strengthening the general health services, standardization through DOTS can jeopardize the very aim of standardizing TB care in the first place, by marginalizing patients from treatment and creating MDR-TB. Many of the authors seem to suggest that the balance between local adaptation and standardization is tilted towards standardization, without leaving enough room, flexibility and capacity to adapt locally. And that less standardization and more elements of individual care and local adaptation are needed. What is more, concerns about increasing drug resistance may reinforce this tilted balance, with stricter forms of supervision, control and standardization as ways to deal with the complexity of detecting and treating highly resistant TB strains.

Standardization and local adaptation in MDR-TB treatment in India

In earlier work we have suggested that this presumed dilemma might be overcome by more attention to how standardization is practised and made to work. The ethnographic accounts of Harper and Isaakidis reveal how much effort and work is involved in localizing and implementing guidelines in ways that respond flexibly to structural factors and patients' needs. Earlier fieldwork on practices for making DOTS Plus work at one of the first MDR-TB treatment sites shows that the nature of both local adaptation and standardization is ambiguous and unstable and that situating standards happens through what we termed recognizing core recommendations (e.g. supervision, duration, DOTS providers) and going beyond guidelines (e.g. nutritional support, extra counselling, home visits) (Engel and Zeiss, 2014). I will briefly discuss these points below.

Standardization and local adaptation are both ambiguous and unstable
Both too much and too little local adaptation, or too much adherence, are risky and problematic. The variant of DOTS that the RNTCP implements does not really reach into the private sector and in rural areas there is not much oversight of how DOTS is practised (Bhatter, Chatterjee and Mistry, 2012). Instead of a database and a comprehensive surveillance system, the RNTCP relied for many years on patient adherence and patient information (Bhatter, Chatterjee and Mistry, 2012). From this perspective the standardization does not go far enough. Yet, at the same time, the guidelines can be too strict to cope with the realities of daily life, and thus adherence can be risky to

individual health and TB control (Engel and Zeiss, 2014). For poor TB patients who lost their jobs when they fell ill or because visits to the DOTS centre were incompatible with work, strictly following the guidelines is impossible. They become hungrier when their health improves, but are unable to afford the food. Patients without a residential address are not eligible for treatment. Only when programme staff adapt the guidelines and draw maps on patients' cards to indicate their makeshift homes do they become eligible for the TB treatment. Yet adapting guidelines can also be detrimental to individual health and TB control if treatment is mismanaged, causing further amplification of drug resistance, if numbers are fudged or if professionals over-rule patients when adapting locally. The nature of both local adaptation and standardization is thus ambiguous (Engel and Zeiss, 2014).

Recognizing core recommendations

In treating patients for TB and MDR-TB, deviation from the guideline happens if the situation requires it. Staff deviate from the guidelines when they draw neighbourhood maps on TB patients' cards to indicate makeshift homes or huts so as to make patients who do not have a residential address eligible for the programme (which otherwise they would not be). Yet, in conversations about these deviations with TB programme staff, clinicians and DOTS providers it became clear that there are certain things that are core to the guidelines and that cannot easily be deviated from. These core recommendations include the drug regimen or direct supervision of patients. An NGO programme manager who works among practitioners and patients explained that collaboration with the public TB programme meant that they had to align their project with the basic principles of DOTS. Distance and the limited opening hours of existing public health facilities often deter patients from taking their treatment regularly. The NGO was able to offer more accessible NGO community DOTS centres with flexible opening hours to increase accessibility, but still needed to ensure that patients were at the facility and supervised when taking their treatment.

> It was not totally free for us to do anything we wished under the project, it had to be within the guidelines of course of the RNTCP. We cannot have a DOTS centre wherein we are giving treatment for a patient for a month because they [the patients] cannot come here. If it is DOTS, it has to be DOTS even in an NGO DOTS centre. (Interview, NGO programme manager 1, 19 December 2009)

Deviating from such core recommendations can happen in exceptional situations, in consultation with superiors. For instance, if a patient needs to travel a physician can, in consultation with superior programme management levels, provide the patient with the drugs for those days. A WHO consultant explains how the recommendation of direct supervision by a trained DOTS provider can be deviated from in exceptional situations:

> For example: there is a situation in the field where there is a hamlet consisting of five houses with nothing within 25km. And you don't find a DOTS provider. You want a family member, but the guidelines don't allow that. The good thing in such a situation, as a WHO consultant you are never an orphan you can call up others [WHO consultants]. You can discuss, they might say, OK, go ahead, and then you ask the STBO [State TB Officer]. These kind of exceptional approvals happen. (Interview, WHO consultant 3, 26 November 2008)

In the practice of applying guidelines, actors reconcile the tension and presumed dilemma between standardization and localization. The guidelines are made to work by assessing the role of guidelines in that particular moment and whether good care or effectiveness is produced in this way (actors define effectiveness differently, see Engel, 2011). Situated assessment of guidelines involves creating a hierarchy within the guidelines of those parts that can be deviated from and other parts that are core recommendations. Core recommendations can be deviated from only in exceptional cases, in consultation with superiors. Situating guidelines in this way differs from deviating too much, such as committing fraud or fudging numbers, which are also common in the health sector in India. Such negative deviation is more common in resource-constrained situations, if necessary capacities and skills are lacking and strict social hierarchies prevail that deter from negotiating these flexibilities when health staff have too little time, skills or resources at hand to adhere to the guidelines.

This finding, that DOT is core, shows how deeply the element of DOT has penetrated into practice. It requires the ability to negotiate flexibilities with superiors, an ability that is hard to come by in a system focused on reaching targets and on strong social hierarchies. It aligns with our observation that most calls in the literature for more flexibility and decentralization in DOTS models seem to suggest that what should be flexible is where and by whom DOT is provided, but the flexibility is not necessarily in non-DOT options (see, for an example, a study from Senegal: Hane et al., 2007).

Going beyond guidelines

Some forms of locally adapting guidelines do not involve deviation from the guidelines. Rather, things are added on, for instance extra support and counselling about how to best embed MDR-TB treatment into a daily routine or diet: 'Any creativity can still be applied with guidelines: They tell you what to do, they normally don't tell you what not to do' (Interview, WHO consultant 3, Hyderabad, 26 November 2008). Going beyond guidelines often requires extra commitment and resources from the staff and it is not always successful in supporting adherence to guidelines. One of the treating senior physicians at the MDR-TB treatment facility where we conducted fieldwork administered around 170 of the daily injections at a patient's home, rather than expecting the patient to come to the health facility, so as to support the patient in adhering to the treatment. Yet the patient was not able to bear the treatment any longer and refused to continue. To the frustration of the physicians, they failed to motivate him to adhere any longer. The clinicians argued for more institutional support with counselling, also by community-based organizations.

Going beyond the guidelines can also mean that patients find it easier to adhere to guidelines. For instance, those patients who received nutritional support at the treatment site found it easier to adhere to the MDR-TB drugs because they could stomach the drugs more easily, deal with side-effects better and did not need to worry about how to pay for the extra food required – because these drugs make you hungry. Medical sociologists and civil society groups have long argued for nutritional support in order to aid recovery from diseases in contexts of heightened risk of malnutrition (Bhatter, Chatterjee and Mistry, 2012; Farmer, 2003; Narayan, 1998). Yet, from a policy perspective, providing nutritional support as part of the TB programme was regarded as unfeasible. Due to the resource-constrained situation in which the TB programme operates, not providing nutritional support was seen as an accepted trade-off between standardized treatment and local adaptation, favouring the former. Nutritional support is now mentioned in the 2016 and 2017 guidelines as part of the treatment support programme for each patient who needs it, possibly in response to the data collected at the first MDR-TB treatment site. Yet, there are still no direct funds available for the nutritional support of outpatients through the programme; instead, health-workers are encouraged to create synergies with other social welfare schemes (Central TB Division, 2016) and to initiate and finance support locally (Central TB Division, 2017).

This example confirms that, even if there is agreement that the key to the success of DOTS is not observation but providing treatment flexibly and combining it with additional support measures, the decentralization of TB care, often viewed as the more flexible and accessible option, works only if the peripheral levels of the health system are supported to go beyond observation (Greene, 2004; Macq et al., 2003). Among doctors, nurses, DOTS providers, NGOs and researchers attending a global TB conference, Macq and colleagues noted more attention to tailoring DOT to local contexts and moving from DOT as supervision of drug intake to DOT as social support (Macq et al., 2003). In DOT as social support the DOTS provider's role was seen as being someone who goes beyond physically observing patients swallowing their drugs, who finds creative ways to make life more acceptable for patients and who, through that, supports them in successfully completing their treatment. This understanding requires more attention to the DOTS provider, their identity within the community and their relations with providers and patients. Providing social support requires someone who is accepted and understood by patients and who can draw on additional emotional and, at times, material resources to support them (Macq et al., 2003). In India DOTS providers are often not well equipped to provide that support and they are seen as supervisors of drug intake more than as social support providers. Going beyond the guidelines and DOTS is difficult if peripheral structures are not strengthened and time and skills are limited to medically trained staff. This will likely remain a challenge, despite increased flexibility for local adaptation in the RNTCP guidelines.

Internalizing guidelines

Situating standards through recognizing core recommendations and going beyond guidelines adds to workload and requires extra skills, capacities, flexibility and sensitivity to different social contexts. The particular control culture of the Indian TB programme – with its strong bureaucratic structure, strong data and target orientation and its approach to centrally implementing tested and proven protocols rather than an approach based on trial and error and continuous learning – has benefits and pitfalls for situating standards through what we termed internalization of guidelines (Engel and Zeiss, 2014). This internalization implies a belief in guidelines and a focus on satisfying guidelines in practice. This was evidenced in the fieldwork by most RNTCP staff, but also by DOTS volunteers and NGO fieldworkers, who revealed a particular focus on data and numbers such as cure and detection rates, treatment categories or numbers of cases on treatment. They had internalized RNTCP talk, thinking and control practices. The focus on the metrics of TB control risks not paying attention, investing in or experimenting with interventions that do not contribute visibly to these numbers or that might negatively impact on the targets, in case new ideas do not work out. The internalization of guidelines is thus an example of the problems with what counts in global health (Adams, 2016). In this way the internalization of guidelines can impede situated standardization. Internalization of guidelines can, however, also foster situating standards. The strong reporting and recording focus of the RNTCP has also been heralded as having added rigour and thereby strengthened the health system. Internalization of guidelines can provide a sense for core recommendations that remain unchanged and for the limits of local adaptation. The promise of situated standardization when having guidelines internalized is to know when and how to adapt locally. The pitfalls are that this level of reflection is omitted as a result of internalizing the guidelines, by which point they are no longer reflected upon (versus the promise that reflection will happen automatically, due to the internalized character) (Engel and Zeiss, 2014).

Conclusion

Much of the existing literature on DOTS argues that, due to the strong medicalization in DOTS, particularly the paternalistic approach to direct observation, the standardization does not do justice to sociocultural contexts and individual care needs, and that, in combination with weak health systems, DOTS is marginalizing, creating defaulters and contributing to MDR-TB. Joanna Crane has emphasized that it is not so much individual pill-taking behaviour that determines resistance patterns, but historical treatment access, markets and politics (Crane, 2013) – and, as discussions around DOTS show, medicalization and standardization of care delivery. In these discussions standardization and local adaptation are often presented as a dilemma. This chapter has highlighted how a focus on how standards are made to work confirms the science and technology studies insight that standardization in TB control is ongoing, localized, emerging, negotiated and based on prior routines and relations. In making standards such as treatment guidelines for tuberculosis work, actors assess the role of guidelines in a particular situation and on that basis recognize the core recommendations of the guidelines or go beyond the guidelines (Engel and Zeiss, 2014). In this way actors negotiate how standards (in this case multi drug resistant treatment guidelines in India) should be situated and, in such situated assessments, they decide when to deviate in order to be effective (Zuiderent-Jerak, 2007a, 2007b). Both standards and the practices wherein they are applied are being shaped by this interaction. As the examples showed, the core recommendations (the local universalities) are being created through localized negotiation between different staff members, the pre-existing relations between them and the routines embedded in the organizational control culture of the TB programme. The application of core recommendations functions as a way to coordinate across the different practices and understandings of different actors.

By negotiating a particular relationship between standardized treatment and the needs of individual care, the actors at the first MDR-TB treatment sites solved a basic public health dilemma between local adaptation and standardization. Qualitative studies on local adaptation can help to specify discussions about what it takes to make guidelines work, can move beyond presumed dilemmas and can play an important role for guideline developers by revealing existing practices in relating to and negotiating local adaptation and standardization.

References

Adams, V. (ed.) (2016) *Metrics: What Counts in Global Health*. Durham, London: Duke University Press.

Agarwal, S. P., Vijay, S., Kumar, P. and Chauhan, L. S. (2005) 'The history of tuberculosis control in India: glimpses through decades', in, *Tuberculosis Control in India*, ed. S. P. Agarwal and L. S. Chauhan (pp. 15–22). New Delhi: Directorate General of Health Services, Ministry of Health and Family Welfare.
Anderson, W. (2006) *The Collectors of Lost Souls. Turning Kuru Scientists into Whitemen*. Baltimore: Johns Hopkins University Press.
Banerji, D. (1998) 'Is TB getting out of hand?', *Indian Journal of Tuberculosis* 45, 180–181.
Bhargava, A., Pinto, L. and Pai, M. (2011) 'Mismanagement of tuberculosis in India: causes, consequences, and the way forward', *Hypothesis* 9 (1), 1–13.
Bhattacharyya, O., Reeves, S. and Zwarenstein, M. (2009) 'What is implementation research? Rationale, concepts, and practices', *Research on Social Work Practice* 19 (5), 491–502.
Bhatter, P., Chatterjee, A. and Mistry, N. F. (2012) 'The dragon and the tiger: realties in the control of tuberculosis', *Interdisciplinary Perspectives on Infectious Diseases* 2012 (Article ID 625459).
Bowker, G. and Star, S. L. (1999) *Sorting Things Out. Classification and Its Consequences*. Cambridge, MA: MIT Press.
Central TB Division (2005) *Technical and Operational Guidelines for Tuberculosis Control*, www.tbcindia.org.
Central TB Division (2010) *RNTCP DOTS Plus Guidelines*, http://tbcindia.org.
Central TB Division (2016) *Technical and Operational Guidelines for Tuberculosis Control in India*, http://tbcindia.gov.in/index1.php?lang=1&level=2&sublinkid=4573&lid=3177.
Central TB Division (2017) *Guidelines on Programmatic Management of Drug-resistant Tuberculosis in India*, https://tbcindia.gov.in/index1.php?lang=1&level=2&sublinkid=4780&lid=3306.
Chakraborty, A. K. (2003) *Expansion of the Tuberculosis Programme in India: Policy Evolution towards Decentralization and Integration*. Pune: The Maharashtra Association of Anthropological Sciences (MAAS).
Conrad, P. (1992) 'Medicalization and social control', *Annual Review of Sociology* 18 (1), 209–232.
Craig, G. M. (2007) '"Nation", "Migration" and Tuberculosis', *Social Theory & Health* 5, 267–284.
Crane, J. (2013) *Scrambling for Africa: AIDS, Expertise, and the Rise of American Global Health Science*. Ithaca and London: Cornell University Press.
Das, J. et al. (2015) 'Use of standardised patients to assess quality of tuberculosis care: a pilot, cross-sectional study', *The Lancet Infectious Diseases* 15 (11), 1305–1313.

Das, V. and Das, R. K. (2006) 'Urban health and pharmaceutical consumption in Delhi, India', *Journal of Biosocial Science* 38 (1), 69–82.

Deshmukh, R. D. et al. (2015) 'Patient and provider reported reasons for lost to follow up in MDRTB treatment: a qualitative study from a drug resistant TB centre in India', *PLoS ONE* 10 (8), e0135802.

Enarson, D. and Billo, N. (2007) 'Critical evaluation of the global DOTS expansion plan', *Bulletin of the World Health Organization* 85 (5), 395–398.

Engel, N. (2011) 'Local adaptation versus standardization? Treatment delivery for multi-drug resistant tuberculosis in India', *Medische Antropologie (Medicine Anthropology Theory)*, 23 (1), 45–61, www.medanthrotheory.org/read/1418/local-adaptation-versus-standardization-treatment-delivery-for-multi-drug-resistant-tuberculosis-in-india.

Engel, N. (2013) 'The making of a public health problem: multi-drug resistant tuberculosis in India', *Health Policy and Planning* 28 (4), 375–385.

Engel, N. (2015) *Tuberculosis in India: A Case of Innovation and Control*. Delhi: Orient Black Swan Ltd.

Engel, N. and Zeiss, R. (2014) 'Situating standards in practices: multi drug-resistant tuberculosis treatment in India', *Science as Culture* 23 (2), 201–225.

Farmer, P. (1997) 'Social scientists and the new tuberculosis', *Social Science & Medicine* 44 (3), 347–358.

Farmer, P. (1998) *Infections and Inequalities. The Modern Plagues*. Berkeley, Los Angeles, London: University of California Press.

Farmer, P. (2003) *Pathologies of Power: Health, Human Rights and the New War on the Poor*. London, Berkeley: University of California Press.

Garner, P. and Volmink, J. (2003) 'Directly observed treatment for tuberculosis: less faith, more science would be helpful', *British Medical Journal* 327 (7419), 823–824.

Greene, J. A. (2004) 'An ethnography of nonadherence: culture, poverty, and tuberculosis in urban Bolivia', *Culture, Medicine and Psychiatry* 28 (3), 401–425.

Hane, F. et al. (2007) 'Identifying barriers to effective tuberculosis control in Senegal: an anthropological approach', *The International Journal of Tuberculosis and Lung Disease* 11 (5), 539–543.

Harper, I. (2005a) 'Anthropology, DOTS and understanding tuberculosis control in Nepal', *Journal of Biosocial Science* 38 (1), 57–67.

Harper, I. (2005b) 'Interconnected and inter-infected: DOTS and the stabilisation of the tuberculosis programme in Nepal', in *The Aid Effect: Giving and Governing in International Development*, ed. D. Mosse and D. Lewis (pp. 126–149). London, Ann Arbor, MI: Pluto Press.

Harper, I. (2010) 'Extreme condition, extreme measures? Compliance, drug resistance, and the control of tuberculosis', *Anthropology & Medicine* 17 (2), 201–214.

Isaakidis, P., Rangan, S., Pradhan, A., Ladomirska, J., Reid, T. and Kielmann, K. (2013) '"I cry every day": experiences of patients co-infected with HIV and multidrug-resistant tuberculosis', *Tropical Medicine & International Health* 18 (9), 1128–1133.
Koch, E. (2016) 'Negotiating "the social" and managing tuberculosis in Georgia', *Journal of Bioethical Inquiry* 13 (1), 47–55.
Lampland, M. and Star, S. L. (eds) (2009) *Standards and Their Stories. How Quantifying, Classifying, and Formalizing Practices Shape Everyday Life*. Ithaca: Cornell University Press.
Lerner, B. H. (1997) 'From careless consumptives to recalcitrant patients: the historical construction of noncompliance', *Social Science & Medicine* 45 (9), 1423–1431.
Lock, M. and Nguyen, V. K. (2010) *An Anthropology of Biomedicine*. West-Sussex, UK: Wiley-Blackwell.
Macq, J. C. M., Theobald, S., Dick, J. and Dembele, M. (2003) 'An exploration of the concept of directly observed treatment (DOT) for tuberculosis patients: from a uniform to a customised approach', *International Journal of Tuberculosis and Lung Disease* 7 (2), 103–109.
Maher, D., Gupta, R., Uplekar, M., Dye, C. and Raviglione, M. (2000) 'Directly observed therapy and treatment adherence', *The Lancet* 356 (9234), 1031–1032.
McDowell, A. and Pai, M. (2016) 'Treatment as diagnosis and diagnosis as treatment: empirical management of presumptive tuberculosis in India', *International Journal of Tuberculosis and Lung Disease* 20 (4), 536–543.
Mykhalovskiy, E., McCoy, L. and Bresalier, M. (2004) 'Compliance/adherence, HIV, and the critique of medical power', *Social Theory & Health* 2 (4), 315–340.
Nagpaul, D. R. (1999) 'An agenda for research in tuberculosis control', *Indian Journal of Tuberculosis* 46, 141–145.
Narayan, T. (1998) *A Study of Policy Process and Implementation of the National Tuberculosis Control Programme in India*. Doctoral dissertation, London: University of London.
Narayan, T. (1999) 'A violation of citizens' rights: the health sector and tuberculosis. One's understanding of the problem of tuberculosis affects the choice of intervention strategies', *Indian Journal of Medical Ethics* 7 (3), 75–78.
Noyes, J. and Popay, J. (2007) 'Directly observed therapy and tuberculosis: how can a systematic review of qualitative research contribute to improving services? A qualitative meta-synthesis', *Journal of Advanced Nursing* 57 (3), 227–243.
Obermeyer, Z., Abbott-Klafter, J. and Murray, C. J. L. (2008) 'Has the DOTS strategy improved case finding or treatment success? An empirical assessment', *PLoS ONE* 3 (3), e1721.

Ogden, J. (1999) 'Compliance versus adherence: just a matter of language? The politics and poetics of public health', in *Tuberculosis: An Interdisciplinary Perspective*, ed. J. M. Grange and J. Porter (pp. 213–234). London: Imperial College Press.

Ogden, J. (2000) 'Improving tuberculosis control – social science inputs', *Transactions of the Royal Society of Tropical Medicine and Hygiene* 94 (2), 135–140.

Ogden, J., Walt, G. and Lush, L. (2003) 'The politics of "branding" in policy transfer: the case of DOTS for tuberculosis control', *Social Science & Medicine*, 57, 179–188.

Petryna, A. (2009) *When Experiments Travel: Clinical Trials and the Global Search for Human Subjects*. Princeton, NJ: Princeton University Press.

Pronyk, P. and Porter, J. (1999) 'Public health and human rights: the ethics of international public health interventions for tuberculosis', in *Tuberculosis: An Interdisciplinary Perspective*, ed. J. M. Grange and J. Porter (pp. 99–120). London: Imperial College Press.

Raviglione, M. C. and Uplekar, M. (2006) 'WHO's new Stop TB strategy', *The Lancet* 367 (9514), 952–955.

Satyanarayana, S. et al. (2015) 'Quality of tuberculosis care in India: a systematic review', *International Journal of Tuberculosis and Lung Disease* 19 (7), 751–763.

Seeberg, J. (2014) 'The event of DOTS and the transformation of the tuberculosis syndemic in India', *Cambridge Anthropology* 32 (1), 95–113.

Timmermans, S. (2015) 'Trust in standards: transitioning clinical exome sequencing from bench to bedside', *Social Studies of Science* 45 (1), 77–99.

Timmermans, S. and Berg, M. (1997) 'Standardization in action: achieving local universality through medical protocols', *Social Studies of Science* 27 (2), 273–305.

Timmermans, S. and Berg, M. (2003) *The Gold Standard. The Challenge of Evidence-Based Medicine and Standardization in Health Care*. Philadelphia: Temple University Press.

Timmermans, S. and Epstein, S. (2010) 'A world of standards but not a standard world: toward a sociology of standards and standardization', *Annual Review of Sociology* 36, 69–89.

Udwadia, Z. F. and Pinto, L. M. (2007) Review series: 'The politics of TB: the politics, economics and impact of directly observed treatment (DOT) in India', *Chronic Respiratory Disease* 4 (2), 101–106.

Udwadia, Z. F., Pinto, L. M. and Uplekar, M. (2010) 'Tuberculosis management by private practitioners in Mumbai, India: has anything changed in two decades?' *PLoS ONE* 5 (8), e12023.

Uplekar, M. and Rangan, S. (1993) 'Private doctors and tuberculosis control in India', *Tubercle and Lung Disease* 74 (5), 332–337.

Volmink, J. and Garner, P. (2007) 'Directly observed therapy for treating tuberculosis', *Cochrane Database of Systematic Reviews* (4).

Walt, G. (1999) 'The politics of tuberculosis: the role of process and power', in *Tuberculosis: An interdisciplinary perspective*, ed. J. D. H. Porter and J. M. Grange (pp. 67–98). London: Imperial College Press.

WHO (2002) *An Expanded DOTS Framework for Effective Tuberculosis Control*. Geneva: World Health Organization.

Williams, G. (2001) 'Holding the patient', *Annals of the New York Academy of Science*, 953b (1), 199–207.

Zeiss, R. (2004) *Standardising Materiality. Tracking Co-constructed Relationships between Quality Standards and Materiality in the English Water Industry*. York: University of York.

Zuiderent-Jerak, T. (2007a) 'Preventing implementation: exploring interventions with standardization in healthcare', *Science as Culture* 16 (3), 311–329.

Zuiderent-Jerak, T. (2007b) *Standardizing Healthcare Practices. Experimental Interventions in Medicine and Science and Technology Studies*. Rotterdam: Erasmus University Rotterdam.

Zwarenstein, M., Schoeman, J. H., Vundule, C., Lombard, C. J. and Tatley, M. (1998) 'Randomised controlled trial of self-supervised and directly observed treatment of tuberculosis', *The Lancet*, 352 (9137), 1340–1343.

3

The not-so-distant past, tuberculosis and the DOTS challenge

Jean-Paul Gaudillière, Christoph Gradmann and Andrew McDowell

Introduction

One way to understand the importance of TB and TB control for the emergence of global health is to look at the history of DOTS. For most, the acronym indicates a double phenomenon. First, it brings to mind 'directly observed therapy, short-course' a chemotherapeutic regimen of multi-drug therapy from the 1970s that reduced the duration of TB treatment from between twelve and eighteen months to between six and eight months. Second, it names a 'universal' TB control strategy supported by WHO, the World Bank and other prominent players of global health initiated in 1994 and dubbed DOTS a year later. Of this strategy, the regimen was one of five elements.

This dual meaning led us to consider the methodological and practical challenges of studying the history of DOTS. How do we introduce this multiplicity of voice and perspective? How can the DOTS strategy's particular history be placed within the larger history of TB and its control since the nineteenth century? How do we situate the history of the DOTS regimen for TB in critical studies of global health where medical anthropology rather than medical history has delivered most analyses?

From an opening discussion of historiographies, anthropologies and methodologies, the chapter moves on to consider two important episodes in such a history: the field trials done by the International Union Against Tuberculosis and Lung Disease (IUATLD) in Tanzania in the 1980s, arguably the most important source of inspiration of DOTS, and the reconfiguration of India's National TB programme in response to DOTS in the early 1990s. Both moments serve to highlight and outline a heuristic challenge of global health history: asymmetrical documentation in which some actors' contributions dominate publications and archival repositories, while other actors occur in the archives as traces reconstructed by a reading against the grain of such documentation, using material collection outside of dedicated archives or interviews that facilitate a critical contextualization of existing archives. In each case we have tried to use our materials as what Arlette Farge calls an 'effective social observatory' (Farge, 2013: 94) that tells stories beyond the scope of the purposes for which they were created.

Global health, the DOTS and the two histories of TB

From its creation in 1994, the TB control strategy known as DOTS (derived from the acronym for one of its five elements, directly observed treatment short-course) has come to dominate global health's management of TB. Renamed StopTB from 2006 and recently EndTB, it is arguably one of the quintessential global health interventions.[1] Today EndTB channels donations by more than 1,600 sponsors into a worldwide TB control campaign. After its creation in 2002 the Global Fund selected TB as one of its three flagship infectious diseases, and campaigns to combat these conditions by raising sponsor money globally (Packard, 2016). Yet the origins of DOTS remain strangely opaque. The landmark WHO report of 1994, which preceded the implementation of the DOTS strategy, points to field trials done by the IUATLD in Tanzania, Malawi and Mozambique (WHO, 1994). This move, however, has been interpreted as a WHO public-relations coup to cover up its previous lack of engagement in the field of TB control (Ogden et al., 2003). A detailed account published by IUATLD in 2009 recounts the organization's long-standing engagement in TB control. This included strengthening national control programmes in Tanzania and other countries like Mozambique or Malawi. The engagement scaled up when the IUATLD's Tanzanian trials were singled out by the World Bank for unsurpassed cost-efficiency in 1991 (Arnadottir, 2009), and subsequently inspired the global control strategy DOTS.

It seems useful to reflect on the place that a yet-to-be-written history of DOTS could occupy the historiography of TB. The historiography of TB is as vast as it is uneven and on the following pages we discuss its main themes as a point of departure for understanding the conditions that shaped the DOTS strategy. The existence of two rather different histories of TB is as striking as it is significant. One history is that of TB as a common infectious disease which was central in the clinical medicine and public health of industrializing countries. In this case, it is a history of success. Classic authors like Francis Barrymore Smith or René Jules Dubos tell the story of the decline of TB since the late nineteenth century, writing of a disease that was essentially controlled by addressing the social and environmental factors driving its epidemic. Also, more contemporary texts considering the North American or European history of TB emphasize the role of social medicine and present us with the picture of a substantial decline that was complete before the arrival of antimicrobial chemotherapies immediately after the Second World War (Dubos and Dubos, 1987; Rosenkrantz, 1994; Smith, 1987). Looking at sanatoria, arguably, provided an interesting expansion of the concept of a social disease (Bryder, 1988; Condrau, 2000). Historians took a critical look at the literary trope of the magic mountain and wrote social science-inspired histories of sanatoria. It did indeed make sense to look at such places as total institutions to or focus on the stigmatization that TB sufferers endured (Bryder et al., 2010; Bynum, 2012).[2] The once magic mountains were now interpreted as mountains of misery, and the discipline patients encountered in sanatoria was not part of their treatment, but a surrogate activity that developed where effective treatment was available (Bryder, 1988; Condrau, 2010). With the demise of sanatoria after the Second World War it seems that historiography lost interest in the recent history of the malady. The arrival of antibiotic chemotherapies immediately after the war seemed to deliver a concluding verdict on the history of TB, and, indeed, except for a brief spike in the immediate post-war years, TB had mostly vanished from industrialized countries.[3]

While TB slipped off the radar in industrialized countries, the condition commenced another career. Around 1950, driven by the availability of chemotherapies and the growing popularity of the BCG vaccine, the disease began its career in international health. However, this connection was not something that historians took notice of before the

1990s. By and large they treated TB as a disease of the past until the late 1980s, when the rise of MDR-TB in connection with HIV raised a big question mark over the narrative of TB's demise. Frank Ryan's 1993 journalistic account, revealing how the battle against TB had been considered won while it was in fact lost (Ryan, 1993) was a wake-up call. It foreshadowed later histories that would examine the revival of TB in high-income countries and the condition's previously ignored international health history. Thus, while TB was addressed by international health from right after the war, histories of these activities were not written before the 2000s. Sunil Amrith first drew our attention to the instance of effective drug therapies and mass vaccination campaigns that led to the erosion of the conceptualization of TB as a social disease (Amrith, 2002, 2004). International health work on TB addressed its control in a way that made social conditions appear less and less important. Famously, the Madras drug trials of 1959, which established the efficacy of outpatient treatment and mass vaccination campaigns in India, were driven by an exaggerated belief in the efficacy of vaccines and relative ignorance of the conditions of their implementation (McMillen and Brimnes, 2010; Valier, 2010). Lynda Bryder spelled out in 2010 that there were now two histories of TB, of which the latter, of international health, a co-epidemic with HIV and drug resistance, should be addressed more vigorously (Bryder et al., 2010). Recently the field has seen a lively development. To name just two examples, Christian McMillen and Nils Brimnes have supplied histories of TB in international health and of the high-modernist, technology-driven spirit that fuelled campaigns (Brimnes, 2016; McMillen, 2015).[4]

So what sources can be consulted with regard to the histories of TB chemotherapies and of DOTS specifically? Fortunately, we have a rich corpus of material provided by participants. The British Medical Research Council (MRC) TB unit, which conducted many of the relevant drug trials from the 1940s to the 1980s, published a synthesis of its work over several decades (Fox et al., 1999); some of the researchers and practitioners associated with the MRC enterprise came together in 2004 for an instructive witness seminar (Christie and Tansey, 2005). While in terms of therapy MRC regimes were essentially the basis of DOTS (see below), IUATLD aimed to put these to work in national TB programmes. The IUATLD published a detailed study of the principles and policies of TB control that describes the Tanzanian trials, on which DOTS came to be modelled (Arnadottir, 2009). Without explicitly juxtaposing the MRC accounts that centre on drugs and the regimens that can be built with them, the IUATLD account highlights the degree to which DOTS is a lot more than short-course drug regimens, involving policies on drug provision, documentation, management, a focus on patient compliance and operational research, in particular. If we add these two books to a number of short historical overviews that have been published by practitioners of DOTS or its successors (Dirlikov et al., 2015; Lienhardt et al., 2012; Raviglione and Pio, 2002; Saltini, 2006), we may conclude that quite a few accounts document birth and development of short-course chemotherapy under direct observation. These accounts tend to focus on drug regimens and health policies. Such policies were developed around 1990 and have been brilliantly analysed by Jessica Ogden (Ogden et al., 2003).

Toward an anthropological history of DOTS

In contrast to the relative paucity of historical work on TB after the Second World War, the disease's redefinition as a problem of developing countries and the recent change of its status in international/global health, anthropologists of medicine have accumulated important studies looking at the policies and practices of TB care in Haiti, Russia and Peru (Farmer, 2001, 2004), South Africa (Erica Dwyer), Georgia (Koch, 2013a, 2013b, 2016), China (Dirlikov, 2015a, 2015b; Dirlikov et al., 2015), Nepal (Harper, 2006, 2010, 2014) and India (Engel, ch. 2 this volume; McDowell and Pai, 2016a, 2016b; McDowell, 2017; Seeberg, 2013, 2014; Venkat, 2016). Perhaps because by the 2000s DOTS had become an unquestioned fact of social life in many countries, anthropologists have been enticed by the challenge of turning DOTS – its emergence and implementation – into a unit of fieldwork and enquiry.

This growing body of work has been extremely successful and exemplifies the merits and benefits of in-depth ethnography with a strong focus on local configurations of action. Considered from a historical perspective on the putative transition from international to global health, the existing anthropology of DOTS makes a series of important points.

First, it shows that DOTS, in spite of being a highly standardized regimen of practices defined within the spaces of global health expertise and associated with transnational actors from WHO to the World Bank, is not only a derivative practice coming from above and imposed on countries, care institutions, individual practitioners and patients. These works examine the multiple adjustments and variations involved in DOTS implementation or, better said, its localization. They reveal that differences are not only a matter of national context (something one might expect, given the intense negotiations and political activities involved in the design of national programmes) but also, and more importantly, the consequences of decisions and improvisations bound to local time and place. As a result, DOTS is not always, nor necessarily, DOTS. DOTS as practice may be juxtaposed with non-standard treatment considered as an appropriate response to patients' needs rather than as bad practice (McDowell in Mumbai, India); it may be closely associated with and depending on non-standard interventions, beginning with the invisible but critical presence of care (Dywer in Tugela Ferry, KwaZulu-Natal); it may be integrated into community-health infrastructures and programmes attending to TB in relation to other diseases, namely HIV (Dwyer, 2014; Engelmann and Kehr, 2015; Kehr, 2012); it may incorporate aspects of TB's social life that are rarely discussed at the international level, to refine the problem of adherence beyond the implementation of patient monitoring (Harper in Nepal and Seeberg in India).

Second, anthropological enquiries shed a bright light on the specificity of the DOTS strategy when compared with other programmes targeting 'global emergencies'. Although TB interventions present many commonalities with the management of other core diseases in global health (malaria and HIV/AIDS), like the centrality of access to drugs, it stands out as a strictly 'vertical' and strongly standardized treatment regimen. There are other major differences as well. One is the massive importance of record keeping and paperwork, a phenomenon which all observers insist upon and that can foster internalized standardization on the part of health care providers, which may get in the way of meeting patients' needs (Engel in this volume).

The paper and computer work linked to DOTS – which includes collecting information about patients, the visits they pay (or do not pay), consultations settings and the pills taken to achieve the norm of observed therapy, among many other indicators – is substantially greater than other 1990s-era disease-control programmes. DOTS as TB intervention also aims at monitoring the activities of medical and non-medical personnel in centres associated with programmes. These ethnographers find the monitoring gaze of DOTS shifting from clinical examination and drug distribution to national laboratories responsible for the bacteriological analysis of resistant cases (Koch, 2011, 2013a). The very significant investments of time and energy required by documentation and monitoring have been central to the legitimation of the DOTS strategy because they are one of global health's responses to the need for proper clinical and epidemiological assessment of treatment results and for the surveillance of various personnel and settings (Harper, 2010; Seeberg, 2014). Managerial surveillance, performance and cost-benefit are therefore major considerations behind these investments in record keeping.

Third, by virtue of their local ethnographies almost all enquiries explore the dilemmas of clinical work under DOTS conditions. Given the strong organizational discourse of DOTS promoters, ethnographies often focus on the problematic relationship between programme design and the inevitable instances of scarcity of resources and improvisation in actual practice. One prominent feature of these works is their focus on the complexity and limits of 'observation' as a response to the problem of treatment failure and mounting resistance. They show a diversity of observational arrangements (Harper, 2006, 2010, 2014) – especially when local personnel consider the question of who should be responsible for a patient's actual ingestion of drugs, or when observation is difficult to implement as consequence of the patient's personal or (less often) clinical situation – and record how non-DOTS treatment paths are maintained and eventually claimed as necessary (Dwyer, 2014; McDowell, 2017). A related source of tensions lies in the changing role of non-clinical personnel, who are both deemed indispensable (there is simply no way to do DOTS relying only on physicians) and plagued by institutionalized hierarchies of expertise.

Last but not least, the mere question of what is a DOTS treatment success has been explored at various levels. Dwyer (2014) follows the ways in which multiple and then extreme drug resistance has become a prominent issue in South Africa in terms of work practices, programme design and the creation of specialized infrastructure for research and care. In contrast, Venkat reveals some of the ways in which the visibility and statistical incidence of multi-drug resistance in India poses questions of DOTS's temporality, reminding us to consider the way DOTS constructs cure from biological uncertainties (Venkat, 2016).

These anthropological enquiries pose two related problems. The first is shared generally by anthropological work. The (classical) centring of ethnography on an embodied researcher creates focuses on 'local' situations of care (within the spaces of community, consultation room, hospital, home) and implies that the construction of DOTS occurs at other levels – often in the specific spaces of global health and in non-medical ways. It leaves more general and contextual ingredients barely investigated per se, for instance political and economic decision making in national, regional and international settings, from country capitals to the World Bank offices in Washington. The second is that of the time gap. Situated in the present, anthropological enquiries have almost uniformly left out of their purview the period of the 1980s and 1990s (except for Farmer, who was writing with the 1990s as the ethnographic present). These decades were decisive in crafting an international consensus on DOTS among global health actors and in starting the first major national programmes (in Tanzania, China and India).

One example clarifies these points. From the vantage point of chronological depth and the impact of economic and political events, the most impressive ethnography of DOTS is Erin Koch's investigation of *Free-market Tuberculosis* in post-Soviet Georgia (Koch, 2013a). Her analysis strongly contrasts the practice of DOTS with the handling of TB during the Soviet era as remembered by her physician informants. DOTS replaced an existing regimen comprising X-ray diagnosis, active case detection, hospital stays and medico-social care including rest and food with the standardized regimen of four drugs, bacteriological diagnosis, passive case finding, ambulatory but observed distribution of drugs and general monitoring. Koch highlights the radical departure in the context of neoliberal policies and an accelerated march toward a market-based economy. DOTS thus came with a reduction in state health spending and a general pattern of structural adjustment aimed at privatizing public industries and services. Rather than taking issue with observation and its disciplinary component, Koch's practitioners target a 'free market' TB that has reduced the clinic to a form of 'primary health care' typical of a 'developing country', while patients caught in a general political and economic crisis try to avoid costs and consultation fees through the direct purchase of antibiotics in local pharmacies. Nostalgia and the dark side of the neoliberal transition are prominent features of DOTS in Georgia, and Koch provides an ethnography laden with history and political economy. However, the past is present only in the form of doctors' memory, while state or global health actors have not been encountered or followed beyond their presence in and impact on the sites of observation.

There is a need for a combined historical and anthropological agenda addressing these two gaps. However, there are serious methodological challenges in launching a historical enquiry into the emergence and changes of DOTS, combining interests in knowledge, practices and policies. The first is a lack of access to archives for the most recent period (basically after 2000), since no institutional archives, from WHO to the World Bank or nation-states, disclose documents less than twenty or thirty years old. A second issue is that such archives, when they are accessible, focus on administration and politics, or on the role of recognized experts, with a paucity of documentation on what researchers, practitioners – not mention patients – have actually done. Finally, the available archives (especially when they have been thoroughly sanitized) often consist of formal records, leaving out visible tensions and (worse) actual decision-making processes, to display the final outcome as consensual and rational.

Writing history in such circumstances may seem a daunting task. However, why should writing the history of DOTS be any easier than contemporary history in general? Historians of the twentieth century have developed responses to similar challenges when documenting the life and actions of workers beyond the role of trade unions and political parties, when attempting to document the trajectories of social movements or when documenting colonial situations from the perspective of subalterns. Three kinds of sources alternative to institutional papers have often been mobilized: (a) interviews following oral history methodologies; (b) collections of privately owned written material; (c) observation of sites and the use of material traces. All of these have proved essential in writing the history of colonial medicine. While historians tend to view oral narratives of the past as a dubious secondary source of data with which to enrich their periodization, add stories or double check archival data, for anthropologists or oral history practitioners they can be used as primary sources of information on the past, examining the ways in which narratives are emplotted around nodes of social meaning and power. Our contention is therefore that all these sources – from conventional archives to oral memories – can be 'read against the grain'.

Tanzania and India: anthropological history and the dialectic of sources

Tanzania and the origins of DOTS
From our perspective, the most interesting story to tell about the Tanzanian National TB and Leprosy Program (NTLP) and its connection to DOTS is one located in a period when nobody even thought of that connection. In the late 1970s global health was not a label for health interventions in the South, and a resurgence of TB in the North was not on the agenda, not to mention its co-epidemic with HIV. It is only in retrospect and in light of its further trajectory that the Tanzanian programme looks like a blueprint case of a global health intervention; hence the need for a cautious analysis of a Tanzania-based IUATLD project that looked anything but innovative at the time of its inception in 1979.

The available documentation on TB control in 1980s Tanzania is rather uneven, mostly consisting of publications, grey literature and some archival material that is almost exclusively connected to the IUATLD and its activities. Thus we have a rich set of reports provided by Union consultants to their organization and its sponsors, and some documentation surviving from the work of the responsible consultant, Karel Styblo.[5] We face a classical situation of archival asymmetry, with traces documenting the activities of institutions in a rather aggregated way, giving voice to international players and promoters of the DOTS strategy, leaving out the involvement of Tanzanian health professionals or issues that tended to be downplayed, like the importance of HIV before 1990. Such material can be and has to be read counter to the grain so as to recover stories that are not the focus of such reports. Such a reading strategy means not only taking the origins and targets of such highly political texts into account; more importantly, it requires considering what uncertainties, difficulties or failures they point to in their own way, and what they remain silent about.

It is also important not to project more recent knowledge about the further history of TB onto an older history. Working on TB control in the 1980s may look timely to us, but it was not for most contemporaries. As a project about a specialized, vertical intervention, the IUATLD's project ran counter to the WHO's policy, which at that time favoured integration of TB control into general health services. In the early 1980s, based on his experience in India, H. Mahler, in his capacity as WHO director general, refused an IUATLD proposal for support and generalization of its Tanzanian experience, arguing that the WHO response to the TB challenge was already in place with the Alma-Ata primary health care strategy.[6] Funding thus came from the Swiss and Dutch governments and not through the WHO. Even the necessity of work on TB as such was not obvious in 1979. After all, African TB seemed to be in slow but steady recession. Successful treatment seemed possible through the application of a large portfolio of treatment regimens developed by MRC researchers from the 1950s to the 1970s. Such work had consisted in the adaption of TB combination therapies, as developed in high-income countries, to their application in developing countries. Some expensive preparations were replaced by cheaper ones and outpatient treatment protocols were developed to serve in places without a sufficient number of hospital beds. Finally, over two decades a steady stream of new preparations facilitated shortening the treatment period from about eighteen months to eight months.

Alas, much of this strategy was paper science in which the sheer existence of working treatment regimens had fostered a sense of complacency. In fact, chemotherapy regimens had gained little traction. In Kenya a 1966 review concluded that only a third of all new cases annually received treatment and only half of these were cured. Effective treatment protocols had hardly been applied outside of trial sites. 'It is really only where the M.R.C. trials are operating or where WHO. has a specific interest that there is much active work being done in tuberculosis at all,' a British researcher remarked in 1964.[7] Prevalence rates were based on screening, but active case-finding, which would have established more reliable numbers and brought more people into treatment, was mostly absent. The existence of chemotherapies suggested a solution that in reality was not put into practice. As a review concluded, 'to rely on chemotherapy of people who present themselves because they have symptoms is a policy which is not likely to reduce tuberculosis'

(Roelsgaard et al., 1964). There is some indication that the development of short-course protocols in the 1970s did little to improve this. In a situation of low treatment completion rates and unsatisfactory adherence to regimens in the first place, it was feared that the implementation of short-course protocols, which required the use of more modern and more expensive drugs, would only add to the problem of drug resistance. Thus, despite the existence of advanced and intricate treatments, in reality 'Monotherapy with isoniazid was the cheap answer to Third World tuberculosis,' as John Crofton concluded in retrospect (Christie and Tansey, 2005).

Against the backdrop of sophisticated trial science that had failed to translate into population-wide control we can understand the innovative character of the IUATLD trials in Tanzania that started in 1979. Employing initially a vintage regimen that combined streptomycin, isoniazid and thiacetazone, the project focused on operational improvements, care and epidemiology to give existing regimens traction throughout the country. Examining what was introduced, we can imagine what was lacking before: systematic reporting of new cases and treatment was introduced; diagnosis through sputum microscopy – rather than X-ray – was made the compulsory standard; drugs were provided free of charge. Hospitalization, having been the Ministry of Health's policy before, although probably insufficiently implemented, was now officially abandoned. In effect, a large number of patients received outpatient treatment upon the programme's inception. This in turn created other challenges. An IUATLD progress report noted that some patients on outpatient treatment, despite living long distances from the nearest health centre, preferred streptomycin injections over their oral replacement, ethambutol.[8]

By 1981 compliance with the defined rules of diagnosis, treatment and reporting seems to have improved. Based on the rich data that was produced, the project's leader, Karel Styblo, an epidemiologist, could now calculate treatment outcomes with a higher degree of precision. While case reporting improved from the start, treatment outcomes started to do so only after the introduction of eight-month short-course regimens and after an initial hospitalization phase of two months was (re)introduced. This approach came to replace the original three-drug, outpatient therapy that had lasted over a year. From 1982 on, a 1970s MRC regimen with four drugs for two months under hospitalization, followed by a six-month outpatient treatment with two drugs, was introduced, resulting in treatment successes of nearly 90%.

Styblo kept an eager eye on the efficiency of the programme. Such efficiency was of course organizational, i.e. choosing the right protocol and building proper institutions, with the consequence that treatment failure would become a problem of individual compliance. In this respect the endeavour did little to end the old blame game that had accompanied anti-infective drug therapies since their invention (Podolsky, 2015). Treatment failure would still be blamed on the non-compliant patient, while social conditions that drive epidemics and complicate therapy fell below the radar. The issue of drug-sensitivity testing was given low priority when developing the NTLP. While diagnostic and treatment capacities with regard to smear-positive cases were greatly expanded, diagnostic facilities in relation to drug-sensitivity testing remained insufficient. In a period when more and more patients came under treatment and the introduction of short-course chemotherapy was supposed to be accompanied by such testing, the country remained stuck with just one functional sputum-culture laboratory throughout the period 1979–88. Consistently, Styblo wrote of patients with drug resistance as people who had mostly themselves to blame. Commenting on such patients in a report, he did not think that the system should be modified in their interest: 'Patients who developed resistance can be considered, by and large, as people with an undue tendency towards irregularity and self-medication.'[9]

Efficiency was not only a problem of epidemiology. It was also a matter of cost and economy. Styblo noted, for instance, that aiming for a cure rate above 90% would disproportionately increase costs, and therefore should be avoided.[10] 'Very little would be gained at a relatively high cost to try to improve a 90% cure rate', he commented in 1988, summing up his experience over one decade of work on the NTLP.[11] Cost-efficiency was thus aimed at before the Tanzanian TB programme was picked up by the World Bank, and such interest resulted in joint publications of Styblo and Christopher Murray, a health economist who is today known as the driving force behind the GBD project and leader of the Institute for Health Metrics and Evaluation, and who in those days worked for Harvard University's Center for Population Studies (Murray et al., 1991a, 1991b). Towards the end of the 1980s and under the influence of health systems analyses, the IUATLD project changed context and became the basis of the DOTS. The World Bank, from 1991, initiated a large-scale trial in China. The WHO, changing course after two decades of relative neglect for TB care, declared TB a global emergency in 1993. It used the IUATLD trials as examples and condensed the approach into the DOTS strategy that it put into practice from 1995.

In retrospect, the sky-rocketing HIV/TB co-epidemic of those years was the backdrop to all this. However, it deserves to be noted that while DOTS was supposed to be an answer to that crisis, comorbidity had not been part of the original problems studied. On the contrary, the IUATLD's work addressed TB as if it existed on its own. No change of opinion seems to have happened when, from 1985, evidence about the presence of HIV cases was mounting. Sudden and sharp increases in cases were observed in some places and antibody screening, when it became available in 1987, indicated a substantial degree of co-infection. The clinical consequences of such co-infection seemed to be dire. A physician running a TB ward in the west of the country reported: 'a high fatality rate during treatment of HIV positive cases. Even the cases that got cured, confirmed by smears and culture do not seem to enjoy their cure from TB for a long time. From several patients we know that they died within half a year from discharge from TB treatment.'[12] Still, when in 1988 Styblo summed up ten years of work on the Tanzanian NTLP he decided to focus on effective and efficient TB control rather than on the emerging co-epidemic that might threaten the approach of having a specialized programme for TB as such. Noting an increase in TB cases since 1985, Styblo commented that 'this was mainly due to improvement of treatment results after the expansion of short course chemotherapy to the entire country rather than AIDS'.[13] It took him several years to acknowledge that this rise in case numbers was the result not of improved reporting but of a growing co-epidemic.

This short overview of the Tanzanian programme in the 1980s is far from complete but it can serve to expand our understanding of the origins of DOTS and, perhaps, global health. Three features stand out. First, the Tanzanian project built on a revival rather than an invention of specialized, vertical health interventions. It was primarily based on (post-)colonial British trial science around TB combination chemotherapy. 'Even though we didn't call it DOTS we were doing DOTS (Christie and Tansey, 2005),'[14] said Janet Darbyshire when assessing the importance of 1970s MRC trials in 2005. Second, there is little precedent for the strict focus on cost-efficiency, which indeed makes the Tanzanian NTLP appear as a prototype of many global health interventions that were yet to come. This fits in with the further fate of the Tanzanian NTLP as an inspiration for what was to become the DOTS. In their joint publications of 1991 Styblo and Murray combined public health epidemiology with economic analysis. Their projected cost-effectiveness of short-course therapy rested not just on curing more patients than standard therapy would, but also on the projected number of deaths averted or treatment costs avoided in future populations (Murray et al., 1991a, 1991b).[15] Third, the innovative character of the Tanzanian programme lay less in strictly medical practices but in what can be summarized as operational improvements such as drug provision, reporting, transport facilities and the like.

India: the reconfiguration of a national programme

The history of India's National Tuberculosis Program (NTP), from its inception in the 1960s until its replacement by a DOTS-based Revised National Tuberculosis Control Program (RNTCP), has been recounted by N. Brimnes (2016). It was the first programme of its sort in developing countries, and during the years when Halfan Mahler led the WHO it played an exemplary role there. Mahler even participated in the early phases of TB research and control initiatives in India. If one wants to appreciate the radical departure that took place during the revision process, some features of the NTP are important to keep in mind. The NTP emerged to a large extent from field experiments by scientists within the newly created National Tuberculosis Institute (NTI) in Bangalore, which started and administered the programme (Jagota, 2000). Through the 1960s the NTI was the main site of epidemiological and operational research on TB in India. The NTP thus focused on diagnosis by X-rays or sputum analysis and access to antibiotics on a voluntary basis, i.e. the 'felt need approach'. The felt need approach meant that TB-affected patients would approach health centres and take care of their treatment themselves (Banerji, 1993b). It was grounded in the work and writings of NTI social scientists who documented patient behaviour and emphasized patients' search for help to argue that patients would engage in the programme if proper infrastructure, accounting for social, familial and cultural constraints of treatment, was provided (Gothi and Baily, 1965; Nagpaul, 1967, 1989). Finally, the NTP was not a vertical programme. Diagnosis and treatment were the tasks of primary health care personnel, so specialized institutions were needed only in urban areas, on the one hand, and for complicated cases and knowledge production, on the other (Jagota, 2000).

From the mid-1970s onward, mounting constraints produced critiques from within. NTI experts regularly documented and lamented problems in drug supply, absence of bacteriological diagnosis, low success rates and a lack of integration into primary health care, with a quasi-absence in rural areas. In the eyes of NTI experts and others, the problems were organizational rather than grounded in the conception and logic of the NTI (Unnikrishnan and Jagannatha, 1989). Although launching DOTS in the 1990s was envisioned as a response to the NTP's problematic status, it was not an internal response. Rather, it was an external 'revision' both in the sense that it was a WHO–World Bank–Government of India initiative and in that its standard bacteriological diagnosis, mandatory drug regime, patient surveillance and meticulous record keeping departed from the grounding principles of the NTP (Khatri and Frieden, 2000, 2002; Kumar, 2005; Narayan, 1999; Ogden et al., 1999).

Investigating the advent of DOTS in India is therefore investigating a rare continuum of actions ranging from Washington, DC and Geneva, to New Delhi and Bangalore, to state and district TB centres, to clinics and homes. Classical institutional archives are useful and their exploration gave us very important and unexpected insights. The World Bank archives in Washington, DC document in many ways the long process of expert visits, pilot studies, financial and political negotiations with New Delhi that preceded the 1997 loan agreement granting India $100 million for its RNTCP.[16] In contrast, Indian institutional archives proved scant, hence our search for participants in the 1990s events and our long and eventually repeated interviews with them.

Visiting Ahmedabad, on a day in January 2017, we look for the office of Dr Dholakia, an economist working at the Indian Institute of Management. Thirty years earlier, Dr Dholakia had mailed to Joel Almeida, head of the research and surveillance unit within the WHO global TB programme, a report entitled 'The potential economic benefits of the DOTS strategy against TB in India' (Dholakia et al., 1997). The report became an official WHO document in 1998, finding its way into both the Geneva and Washington, DC (World Bank) archived files on TB and several libraries in India. As an economic assessment of DOTS, this was an intriguing text, both because of its mere existence (there are few economic studies of global health projects) and because it did not make a single allusion to DALYS, then the most important WHO–World Bank tool of medico-economic evaluation. Dr Dholakia soon explained: 'The whole purpose of this exercise, it is not finding out if it is a question of cost (...) [it was] to compare the two alternatives and what are the benefits and if one is superior to the other, then (...) what is the maximum I can spend to incentivize the people so that this succeeds.'

Thus he restated the report's executive summary, namely that it was not about assessing the feasibility of DOTS following the method central to health economics, i.e. costs/benefits balancing. It was an opposite move: quantifying the economic output of DOTS in order to check economic (not technical) feasibility. Insisting on his computation of output on a 'labour productivity' basis, Dr Dholakia explained:

> The method that I took is a different type of things. It was a substitute of the DALY. It was not a question of the quality of life that the patient undergoes. (...) Say for instance if you are suffering from TB you would not be in a position to attend a full-time job. So you would necessarily be sick on certain days and, you know, you would not be able to do that so what is that kind of proportion.

Dholakia was not a health economist and explained that he knew little about health in general and TB in particular when he was approached to conduct the assessment. According to him (and nothing contradicts that in the WHO archives) that was precisely the reason why Almeida looked for him. He could look at DOTS from the perspective of a development economist. His calculation of the benefits of DOTS thus rested on the evaluation of the labour 'productivity' lost because patients could not work. The first step was to disentangle average productivity:

> Productivity is not [available]. (...) Like say for instance in India we have the estimates of rural and urban income made separately. If at the national level you have urban and rural income estimated separately then I use that to get urban productivity and rural productivity. Then from there I say: ok, what about the sex thing. I made use of an old thesis on sources of economic growth and they had estimated the quality of labour with a sex division so I used some multipliers from there to estimate this thing.

The productivity data were combined with epidemiological data concerning the distribution of TB patients by age, sex and location to compute economic losses due to premature death. The most significant feature was, as he said, that 'patients are not so much concentrated in the age groups of the say 0 15 or 19 because that 15 to 34 and 35 to 59 are the more productive'. The comparison with a complete national implementation of DOTS rested on assumptions about treatment outcomes, case-detection and success rates that Dholakia received from his contact at WHO. They were, unsurprisingly, those used in the promotion of DOTS. Leaving out all considerations of real-life feasibility, this was conscious optimization:

> I was not worried about whether DOTs was implemented and what was the experience on the ground (…) they might have all sorts of problems (…) I did not bother because my only thing was look at the benefits that this particular strategy has a potential to offer; actual practice could be very different because you have not been in a position to provide that kind of a ground or that kind of environment where it will succeed.

This absence of cost and implementation considerations contrasted with what puzzled us in the report, namely the problem of multiple 'discount rates' used to evaluate the impact of diverting investments for DOTS on national growth. Dholakia justified this:

> Because people may not agree (…) If you take a very low discount rate it means that you are actually saying that from the society's point of view the cost of the opportunity cost of capital or of the investment is not very high. (…) There are others who would be arguing that no, no, no, cost of capital is important and we should really consider it as very high, 8 to 9%. You know the planning commission was then talking about 9% and 10%.

Although dealing with TB's impact as well as being commissioned and circulated by the WHO, the study was clearly not that of an economist of health. It was – something impossible to fully appreciate from its reading – targeting specialists in labour and development, the Planning Commission policy makers at the highest level where choices are made regarding investments in dams or dispensaries, hence its circulation within the World Bank headquarters.

Dholakia's interview then resonated with other interviews which we conducted on the preparation of the famous 1993 World Bank report 'Investing in health', which echoed and legitimized the rapid growth of health-related loans in the Bank's activities. These were scant allusions about the tensions between general economists and health economists; the former seeing the development of the DALYs and their use in the first GBD as a 'physicians' tool' rather than economic modelling for public investments.

Meeting Dholakia and discussing his report not only brought new information about the actors or events associated with its production or framing, it also pointed to a very significant divergence between epidemiology, health economics and general economics when assessing the feasibility and usefulness of DOTS. The interview changed the meanings which we attributed to the text when reading it from the perspective of the WHO archives and revealed a critical uncertainty around what kind of econometric thinking ought be brought to bear on health: an economics of development, an economics of performance, or not economics but instead a combination of epidemiology and operations research.

Banerji and documenting 'visions'

Debaber Banerji was the first sociologist embedded within India's nascent National Tuberculosis Institute. Traces of Banerji are manifold. His published works championing a 'felt need approach to TB intervention' are scattered through 1960s TB literature and institutes in India, particularly Jawaharlal Nehru University's Centre of Social Medicine and Community Health archives. At the same time, other sources of history like the WHO's archive in Geneva, the World Bank's archive or the Swedish International Development Agency archive reveal a short correspondence or no sign of Banerji at all. From these sources it would be possible to conclude that Banerji had very little to do with TB initiatives after 1970, and even less to say about them.

Yet in 1993 he responded to India's WHO and World Bank-led revision of the TB programme with an article in *Economic and Political Weekly*. This article, titled 'Simplistic approach to health policy analysis: World Bank team on Indian health sector' (Banerji, 1993a), along with his many other publications, lays out Banerji's key objection to the

World Bank's intervention in Indian health care. He begins by outlining the Bank's five-week visit to review the India TB programme and the report it produced. He writes,

> Indeed, based on a 'vigorous' discussion at a meeting of 'India's most eminent health policy researchers, chaired by the Secretary of Health', the team claims that the report in many ways is a joint statement of the two sides. It is worthy of note that a substantial majority of those who attended the meeting were not even acquainted with some of the basic literature concerning growth and development of public health practice in India, not to speak of health policy research with its political, administrative, technological, epidemiological and sociological dimensions. (Banerji, 1993a: 1207)

He goes on to outline the complexity of a health system, reminds readers of the need for interdisciplinary analyses of health systems and examines the report for what he calls the simplistic perspective that health finance may be the only necessary adjustment to India's health care system. He finishes with another incisive pair of sentences:

> Health financing is one component of health economics, which, in turn, is a component of the wider field of health systems research which is based on inter-disciplinary studies to optimize the highly complex health services system or its smaller components. This 'upside down' study has led the team to advocate a lacerating vivisection of a live organization which has been so painstakingly nurtured and built up over more than six decades. (Banerji, 1993a: 2010)

From this springboard, Banerji published papers considering the importance of operations research in the NTP and entreated readers to oppose a vertical programme for TB (Banerji, 1993b, 1997, 1999, 2002, 2003, 2012). Yet it remained unclear how a man so seemingly committed to providing services for the poor would support a programme that had struggled to care for the few people who accessed it.

To answer this question we visited Banerji in his Delhi home. The day-long, free-wheeling conversation was often structured or emplotted by Banerji's comparison between what he viewed as a Buddhist and democratic political theology and a Christian authoritarian one. Again and again Banerji counterpoised an abiding concern for asking people what they need and what he viewed as an interventionist Christian political theology. By focusing on Banerji's political claims, we add nuance to what might have easily been read as a commitment to primary health care approaches of the 1970s or post-colonial resistance to intervention. Although both are part of the picture, our discussion revealed more.

Discussing the integration of sociology, he suggested:

> I went to NTI because of my commitment to the people and a sociologist is how they accepted me. They had to accommodate me. I said 'what is the sociologist to do?' He [Mahler] said 'well,' almost casually you know, 'the original idea was Holm's', Johannes Holm, he was a Dane too. 'We wanted Johannes to train people to accept the drug and then by various colours and this and that to make it acceptable'; again an example of the Christian saving the heathens in a national way. So this whole idea it was very vague.

However, Banerji did something different from what he considered to be an imposed biomedical approach. Instead, Banerji and his colleagues designed studies of patients' health trajectories to understand how patients were affected by TB and what they did about it. They revealed that 70% of patients noticed TB symptoms and 50% sought biomedical attention at least once before diagnosis. The NTI designed an intervention with this action-taking in mind. This integration of patient perspectives and intervention characterized NTI's felt need approach and what Banerji called a social integration of technology, rather than an interventionist, top-down approach. When Banerji and his colleagues found that people accessed their local health centre, this posed another problem,

> There was a tremendous pressure on India to go for mass radiography and when you catch the people. Catch, like catching mice. Then you have to treat them and to do that they can take the pills brought in by the saviours, they had to save the fellows you know, I'm again using that language, and there were strong supporters of x-ray in 1960 (...) so they said, you know these saviours, they said 'no, no, no, we will give you eight', but somehow, I was a little doubtful that this would fix it, and that is the central sociological contribution, so we tested that with our data.

Instead, Banerji advocated that a 'felt need' programme would let people come to the health system. To do so Banerji needed the microscope, a technology that could be used in local health centres.

It became clear that what seemed like Banerji's conservative perspective on DOTS in 1993 was actually a political theology pushing against what he considered to be the cost-effective and paternalistic moral imperatives built into global health. In his case, the ideal politics is a pragmatic, holistic and democratic health policy that can respond to the political theology of saviourship underpinning the 'verticalization' and the claims of emergency around TB in the 1990s. The revision of the TB programme and its politics highlight, for Banerji at least, the replacement of a political imperative of health decisions made on the basis of democratic citizenship by the moral imperatives of cost-effective charity. By responding to reforms in favour of the existing system Banerji saw himself as working to inject politics into what often appears a depoliticizing or anti-politics reform. Seen from this perspective, Banerji's misrecognized conservativism provides an Indian actor's perspective on what health development and politics might be and throws the contested nature of TB intervention into stronger relief. This diversity of perspective sometimes falls away in histories that rely heavily on Western archives and actors, as Brimnes does to great effect (Brimnes, 2016).

At the same time, there is a modicum of what Koch called nostalgia in Banerji's interview. Although not the nostalgia for a once-implemented Soviet state and health system, Banerji's nostalgia is for a democratic health system and the Nehruvian moment's seemingly endless development possibilities which inspired the felt need approach. He lamented the loss of hope for a state capable of, at least some day, responding to the needs of citizens. Banerji reveals the important links between the NTP and its revisions, the Indian state and what development could be that are echoed somehow in Dholakia's hope for future possibilities.

The multiple moves back and forth between oral testimonies and existing written material, or the fact that many interviews led to the discovery of unknown and valuable documents that our informants kept, open a new way of thinking about connectivity. The connectivity we highlight here is not just across space but also between document and memory, global and local, aspiration and event. The connectivity between two seemingly polar opposite people and perspectives becomes clear only when locating written texts within personal trajectories and institutional debates and tracking back and forth between contemporary and historical interpretation. They are working through similar questions, but in doing so reveal the global health moment's inversion of the relationship between not just the state and the development but health and the economy. For Banerji and the Nehruvian state, developments like dams would create resources that could then be used to address health as people demanded it. Dholakia's report, however, inverts the paradigm to suggest that investments in health generate growth factors or human capital, so what is now needed is not dams but schools and hospitals. At another scale, they track an inversion in what efficiency might mean, as Banerji's modernist perspective held that efficiency ought to be clinical, while Dholakia imagined a global health in which efficiency might be measured in economic effects.

By thinking about other sources of historical data in the context of archival asymmetries – characterized in the Indian case by scarcity – we realized that DOTS' arrival and integration in India was a crucible of conversations broader than TB treatment. We see that although the TB treatment given to millions was now in flux there were other questions about development, action and evidence attached to this change. We learn that DOTS' introduction in India represented a sea-change in thinking about how to guide health care and development, and we uncover the important ways through which existing TB institutions and actors reacted to changes in knowledge and practice coming – to a large extent – from outside their domain of expertise.

Conclusion

The further history of the DOTS strategy is not the subject of this chapter, but from the knowledge we have we can infer that the further development of the DOTS was influenced by certain initial shortcomings that were present in these years: its relative neglect of drug resistance, its reluctance to deal with the TB and HIV co-epidemic, and the degree of suspicion with which it met patients and communities.[17]

The two cases show strong parallels in terms of pointing to continuity, the rise of economics and organizational innovation. However, we are dealing with two different periods and contexts – first, experimentation and the scaling up of the MRC trial science into a nationwide programme, and second, implementation in a context of globalization and the work to fit DOTS into a struggling but extant TB programme. Our treatment of this difference has methodological consequences in terms of what is to be understood about DOTS and how. The 'how', of course, is about reading archives against the grain, on the one hand, and doing oral history at the crossroads of anthropology and history, on the other. In terms of 'what', the Tanzanian case tells us about the intellectual trajectories and experimental practices that coalesced to make of the DOTS strategy, whereas in India DOTS arrived as a finished product and sheds light on the political economy of global TB control.

Together the two cases reveal that one can write an account of global health that crosses scales from a local into the global and back again. Here the focus is on scaling up and down or on local and global movements of a broadened set of entities that include texts, people and practices. By following this game of scales it is possible to write a history and anthropology of global health that takes the local and contingent seriously while connecting them to global processes like economics and epidemics, politics and pharmaceuticals. It becomes clear that local actors cross scales to the global and global actors cross scales to the local, and that this scalability can be studied. Focusing on DOTS with scales in mind, we show that everyone is playing the game of scales, but not in the same way and not with the same ability to generalize.

Notes

1 For a quick overview: WHO, Implementing the End TB Strategy: the Essentials, 2015 (www.who.int reference: WHO/HTM/TB/2015.31)
2 A good overview Bynum (2012).
3 For a summary: Mercer (2014). For an overview of chemotherapies: Greenwood (2008).
4 Cf. Margaret Jones on Sri Lanka. Jones (2016).
5 Tanzania National Tuberculosis / Leprosy Programme: Progress reports no. 1 through 37 [twice annually] by the IUATLD. Courtesy of Hans Rieder, Kirchlindach.
6 A. Rouillon to H. Mahler, 23 November 1982; H. Mahler to A. Rouillon, 21 April 1983. WHO Archives, Geneva, Relations with IUATLD, T9/348–2, Jacket 3.
7 UK Public Record Office, FD 12/554, p. 7 [94].
8 'Report of Visit to Tanzania by Dr K. Styblo and J. A. Sobotkiewicz', January 1979 [International Union Against Tuberculosis Tanzania, report No 1].
9 IUATLD progress reports [as above], No. 3, p. 8.

10 Progress report, 'Results of the NTLP after the First Ten Years', CERMES3, Styblo papers, June 1988.
11 Progress report, 'Results of the NTLP after the First Ten Years', CERMES3, Styblo papers, June 1988.
12 Dekker to Chum, 1988, CERMES3, Styblo papers 1988.
13 Progress report 'Results of the NTLP after the First Ten Years', CERMES3, Styblo papers, June 1988.
14 The comment made on the occasion of a witness seminar was immediately met with the criticism (by D. Mitchison) that the other four elements of DOTS were all but missing in the 1970s trials.
15 The argument for a high number of deaths averted is that effective treatment with short-course therapy in the present changes the epidemic trend and results in less cases to treat in the future. This also explains the focus on smear-positive cases that contribute more to transmission of the disease.
16 World Bank, *Staff Appraisal Report India Proposed Tuberculosis Control Project*, Report no. 15894-IN, 6 January 1997.
17 For critical evaluations of DOTS see Harper, 2010: 201–214 and McMillen, 2015: ch. 12. An overview of following development can be found in Dirlikov, Raviglione and Scano, 2015: 52–58.

References

Amrith, S. (2002) *Plague of poverty? The World Health Organization, tuberculosis and international development, c. 1945–1980*. Cambridge: University of Cambridge.

Amrith, S. (2004) 'In search of a "magic bullet" for tuberculosis: South India and beyond, 1955–1965', *Social History of Medicine* 17 (1), 113–130.

Arnadottir, T. (2009) *Tuberculosis and Public Health: Policy and Principles in Tuberculosis Control*. Paris: IUATLD.

Banerji, D. (1993a) 'Simplistic approach to health policy analysis – World Bank team on Indian health sector', *Economic and Political Weekly* 28 (24), 1207–1210.

Banerji, D. (1993b) 'A social science approach to strengthening India's National Tuberculosis Programme', *Indian Journal Tuberculosis* 40, 61–82.

Banerji, D. (1997) *Serious Implications of the Proposed Revised National Tuberculosis Control Programme for India*. New Delhi: Voluntary Health Association of India and Nucleus for Health Policies and Programmes.

Banerji, D. (1999) 'A fundamental shift in the approach to international health by WHO, UNICEF, and the World Bank: instances of the practice of "intellectual fascism" and totalitarianism in some Asian countries', *International Journal of Health Services* 29 (2), 227–259.

Banerji, D. (2002) 'Report of the WHO Commission on Macroeconomics and Health: a critique', *International Journal of Health Services* 32 (4), 733–754.

Banerji, D. (2003) 'Reflections of an Indian scholar', *International Journal of Health Services* 33 (1), 163–169.

Banerji, D. (2012) 'The World Health Organization and public health research and practice in tuberculosis in India', *International Journal of Health Services* 42 (2), 341–357.

Brimnes, N. (2016) *Languished Hopes. Tuberculosis, the State and International Assistance in Twentieth-Century India*. New Delhi: Orient Black Swan.

Bryder, L. (1988) *Below the Magic Mountain: A Social History of Tuberculosis in twentieth-Century Britain*. Oxford: Clarendon Press.

Bryder, L., Flurin, C. and Worboys, M. (2010) 'Tuberculosis and its histories: then and now', in *Tuberculosis Then and Now: Perspectives on the History of an Infectious Disease*, ed. F. Condrau and M. Worboys (pp. 3–23). Montreal: McGill-Queens University Press.

Bynum, H. (2012) *Spitting Blood: The History of Tuberculosis*. Oxford: Oxford University Press.

Christie, D. A. and Tansey, E. M. (eds) (2005) *Short-Course Chemotherapy for Tuberculosis*. London: The Wellcome Trust Centre for the History of Medicine at UCL.

Condrau, F. (2000) *Lungenheilanstalt und Patientenschicksal. Sozialgeschichte der Tuberkulose in Deutschland und England im späten 19. und frühen 20. Jahrhundert*. Göttingen: Vandenhoeck und Ruprecht.

Condrau, F. (2010) 'Beyond the total institution: towards a reinterpretation of the tuberculosis sanatorium', in *Tuberculosis Then and Now: Perspectives on the History of an Infectious Disease*, ed. F. Condrau and M. Worboys (pp. 72–99). Montreal: McGill-Queens University Press.

Dholakia, R., WHO Global TB Programme (Alemeida, J. and 1997) *The Potential Economic Benefits of the DOTS Strategy Against TB in India*. Geneva: World Health Organization.

Dirlikov, E. (2015a) 'BRICS health and tuberculosis control collaborations during an era of global health', *Medicine Anthropolog, Theory* 4 (2), 136–153.

Dirlikov, E. (2015b) *Controlling Tuberculosis Then and Now: Chinese Public Health Policymaking and Problematizations in an Era of Global Health*. Montreal: McGill University Libraries.

Dirlikov, E., Raviglione, M. and Scano, F. (2015) 'Global tuberculosis control: toward the 2015 targets and beyond', *Annals of Internal Medicine* 163 (1), 52–58.

Dubos, R. J. and Dubos J. (1987 [1952]), *Tuberculosis, Man, and Society*. New Brunswick and New York: Rutgers University Press.

Dwyer, E. C. 'The making of a global health crisis: extensively drug resistant tuberculosis and global science in rural South Africa', Ph.D. thesis, University of Pennsylvania.

Engelmann, L. and Kehr, J. (2015) 'Double trouble? Towards an epistemology of co-infection', *Medicine Anthropology Theory* 4 (2), 1–31.

Farge, A. (2013) *The Allure of the Archives*. New Haven, CT: Yale University Press.

Farmer, P. (2001) *Infections and Inequalities: The Modern Plagues*. Berkeley: University of California Press.

Farmer, P. (2004) *Pathologies of Power: Health, Human Rights, and the New War on the Poor*. Berkeley: University of California Press.

Fox, W., Ellard, G. and Mitchison, D. (1999) 'Studies on the treatment of tuberculosis undertaken by the British Medical Research Council Tuberculosis Units, 1946–1986, with relevant subsequent publications', *International Journal of Tuberculosis and Lung Disease* 3 (10), S231–279.

Gothi, G. and Baily, G. (1965) 'Problems of treatment of tuberculous patients in rural areas', *Indian Journal of Tuberculosis* 12, 62.

Greenwood, D. (2008) *Antimicrobial Drugs. Chronicle of a Twentieth Century Triumph*. Oxford: Oxford University Press.

Harper, I. (2006) 'Anthropology, DOTS and understanding tuberculosis control in Nepal', *Journal of Biosocial Science* 38 (1), 57–67.

Harper, I. (2010) 'Extreme condition, extreme measures? Compliance, drug resistance, and the control of tuberculosis', *Anthropology & Medicine* 17 (2), 201–214.

Harper, I. (2014) *Development and Public Health in the Himalaya: Reflections on Healing in Contemporary Nepal*. London: Routledge.

Jagota, P. (2000) *Annals of the National Tuberculosis Institute*. Bangalore: The Institute.

Jones, M. (2016) 'Policy innovation and policy pathways: tuberculosis control in Sri Lanka, 1948–1990', *Medical History* 60, 514–33.

Kehr, J. (2012) 'Blind spots and adverse conditions of care: screening migrants for tuberculosis in France and Germany', *Sociology of Health & Illness* 34 (2), 251–265.

Khatri, G. R. and Frieden, T. (2000) 'The status and prospects of tuberculosis control in India', *International Journal of Tuberculosis and Lung Disease* 4 (3), 193–200.

Khatri, G. R. and Frieden, T. (2002) 'Rapid DOTS expansion in India', *Bulletin of the World Health Organization* 80 (6), 457–463.

Koch, E. (2011) 'Local microbiologies of tuberculosis: insights from the Republic of Georgia', *Medical Anthropology* 30 (1), 81–101.
Koch, E. (2013a) *Free Market Tuberculosis: Managing Epidemics in post-Soviet Georgia*. Nashville: Vanderbilt University Press.
Koch, E. (2013b) 'Tuberculosis is a threshold: the making of a social disease in post-Soviet Georgia', *Medical Anthropology* 32 (4), 309–324.
Koch, E. (2016) 'Negotiating "the social" and managing tuberculosis in Georgia', *Journal of Bioethical Inquiry* 13 (1), 47–55.
Kumar, P. (2005) 'Journey of tuberculosis control movement in India: National tuberculosis programme to revised national tuberculosis control programme', *Indian Journal of Tuberculosis* 52, 63–71.
Lienhardt, C. et al. (2012) 'Global tuberculosis control: lessons learnt and future prospects', *National Review of Microbiology* 10 (6), 407–416.
McDowell, A. (2017) 'Mohit's Pharmakon: symptom, rotational bodies, and pharmaceuticals in rural Rajasthan', *Medical Anthropology Quarterly* 31 (3), 332–348.
McDowell, A. and Pai, M. (2016a) 'Treatment as diagnosis and diagnosis as treatment: empirical management of presumptive tuberculosis in India', *International Journal of Tuberculosis and Lung Disease* 20 (4), 536–543.
McDowell, A. and Pai, M. (2016b) 'Alternative medicine: an ethnographic study of how practitioners of Indian medical systems manage TB in Mumbai', *Transactions of the Royal Society of Tropical Medicine and Hygiene* 110 (3), 192–198.
McMillen, C. (2015) *Discovering Tuberculosis: A Global History, 1900 to Present*. New Haven: Yale University Press.
McMillen, C. and Brimnes, N. (2010) 'Medical modernization and medical nationalism: resistance to mass tuberculosis vaccination in postcolonial India, 1948–1955', *Comparative Study of Society and History* 52 (1), 180–209.
Mercer, A. (2014) *Infections, Chronic Disease, and the Epidemiological Transition*. Rochester: University of Rochester Press.
Murray, C. J., Styblo, K. and Rouillon, A. (1991a) 'Tuberculosis in developing countries: burden, intervention and cost', *Bulletin International Union Tuberculosis* 65 (1), 6–24.
Murray, C. et al. (1991b) 'Cost effectiveness of chemotherapy for pulmonary tuberculosis in three sub-Saharan African countries', *The Lancet* 338 (8778), 1305.
Nagpaul, D. R. (1967) 'District tuberculosis control programme in concept and outline', *Indian Journal of Tuberculosis* 14 (4), 186–98.
Nagpaul, D. R. (1989) 'India's National Tuberculosis programme – an overview', *Indian Journal of Tuberculosis* 36, 205–11.

Narayan, T. (1999) 'A violation of citizens' rights: The health sector and tuberculosis', *Issues in Medical Ethics* 7 (3), 75–78.

Ogden, J., Walt, G. and Lush, L. (2003) 'The politics of "branding" in policy transfer: the case of DOTS for tuberculosis control', *Social Science & Medicine* 57 (1), 179–188.

Ogden, J. et al. (1999) 'Shifting the paradigm in tuberculosis control: illustrations from India', *International Journal of Tuberculosis and Lung Disease* 3 (10), 855–861.

Packard, R. (2016) *A History of Global Health: Interventions into the Lives of other Peoples*. Baltimore: Johns Hopkins University Press.

Podolsky, S. (2015) *The Antibiotic Era: Reform, Resistance, and the Pursuit of Rational Therapeutics*. Baltimore: Johns Hopkins University Press.

Raviglione, M. C. and Pio, A. (2002) 'Evolution of WHO policies for tuberculosis control, 1948–2001', *The Lancet* 359 (9308), 775–80.

Roelsgaard, E., Iversen, E. and Bløcher, C. (1964) 'Tuberculosis in Tropical Africa', *Bulletin of the World Health Organization* 30, 459–518.

Rosenkrantz, B. (1994) *From Consumption to Tuberculosis: A Documentary History*. New York; London: Garland Publishers.

Ryan, F. (1993) *The Forgotten Plague: How the Battle Against Tuberculosis Was Won – and Lost*. Boston: Little, Brown.

Saltini, C. (2006) 'Chemotherapy and diagnosis of tuberculosis', *Respiratory Medicine* 100 (12), 2085–2097.

Seeberg, J. (2013) 'The death of Shankar: social exclusion and tuberculosis in a poor neighbourhood in Bhubaneswar, Odisha', in *Navigating Social Exclusion and Inclusion in Contemporary India and Beyond: Structures, Agents, Practices*, ed. U. Skoda, K. B. Nielsen, and M. Q. Fibiger (pp. 207–226). London: Anthem Press.

Seeberg, J. (2014) 'The event of DOTS and the transformation of the tuberculosis syndemic in India', *The Cambridge Journal of Anthropology* 36 (2), 95–113.

Smith, F. (1987) *The Retreat of Tuberculosis 1850–1950*. London: Croom Helm.

Unnikrishnan, K. P. and Jagannatha, P. S. (1989) *Performance of National Tuberculosis Programme*. Bangalore: ICORCI.

Valier, H. (2010) 'At home in the colonies: the WHO-MRC trials at the Madras chemotherapy centre in the 1950s and 1960s', in *Tuberculosis then and now: Perspectives on the History of an Infectious Disease*, ed. F. Condrau and M. Worboys (pp. 213–234). Montreal: McGill-Queens University Press.

Venkat, B. (2016) 'Cures', *Public Culture* 28 (3), 475–497.

WHO (1994) *TB: A Global Emergency*. Geneva: WHO.

4

Decolonizing, nationalizing and globalizing the history of psychiatry: from colonial to cross-cultural psychiatry in Nigeria[1]

Matthew M. Heaton

Introduction

While still a relatively nascent field, the historical study of global health in Africa has tended to define its main characteristics in terms of the neoliberalization of the public health landscape in since the 1980s, with a particular emphasis on targeted interventions against infectious diseases, most notably HIV (Langwick, Dilger and Kane, 2012; Prince, 2013). These narratives see historical continuity between colonial and tropical medical structures that used African spaces as 'laboratories' (Keller, 2007; Tilley, 2011) and the international programmes of the WHO that contributed to the modernization schemes of post-colonial African states (Hodge, 2007). Indeed, for James Webb and Tamara Giles-Vernick, who edited the first book-length historical study of global health in Africa, the term 'global health' refers specifically and exclusively to 'the health initiatives launched within Africa by actors based outside of the continent' (Webb and Giles-Vernick, 2013: 3) and focuses heavily on campaigns against infectious diseases since the end of the Second World War.

The question of where mental health fits into this history has yet to be addressed; however, the examination of psychiatry provides a variety of opportunities to complicate the historical narrative of global health in Africa that has been proffered so far. As with other medical sciences, the history of psychiatry in Africa is intimately connected to the processes of European colonialism. A small but coherent historiography has done a great deal to demonstrate the ways that European ideas about mental illness and how to treat it were deeply invested in the racist and paternalistic ideologies of European imperialism in the early twentieth century (Bell, 1991; Deacon, 1996; Jackson, 2005; Keller, 2007; McCulloch, 1995; Sadowsky, 1999; Vaughan, 1983). And it was these structural influences of European racism and colonialism on the colonized psyche that inspired the anti-colonial critiques of Frantz Fanon (1967, 1978). But how do we get from these colonial and anti-colonial contexts to a global history of mental health care that incorporates post-colonial spaces and actors?

This chapter offers a particular context within which to fill the gap between colonial and contemporary global health agendas in the history of psychiatry through an examination of the development of 'modern' mental health services in Nigeria between the 1950s and 1970s. In doing so I hope to de-emphasize the implicit binary that the existing historical narrative constructs between the 'African' and the 'global' – in which the 'global' acts and the 'African' reacts – to show how complex relationships between the local, national and global have framed developments in the field of mental health research and practice both in Nigeria and internationally since the 1950s. Focusing on the life and work of Thomas Adeoye Lambo, Nigeria's first European-trained psychiatrist of indigenous background, the chapter illustrates how the development of mental health services in Nigeria connected to local cultural expectations, nationalist developmentalist agendas and international programmes in cross-cultural psychiatric research over the period from the 1950s to 1970s. Lambo ultimately helped to cement a mental health care paradigm originating from the global North, in Nigeria, in ways that significantly expanded upon the colonial model. However, at the same time he adapted that paradigm to better fit local circumstances, and those adaptations in turn recirculated into the global discourse, affecting the way psychiatrists around the world thought about the nature and treatment of mental illness. The development of mental health infrastructure in Nigeria was therefore local, national and international.

This chapter builds upon recent research in the history of psychiatry that has already begun complicating the use of binary constructions and the notion that international science tends to serve 'external' masters in colonial spaces. For example, recent comparative work in the history of psychoanalysis has shown how the construction of a universal self has had significant global impact, but in diverse ways depending on the local context in which it has been employed. Psychoanalytic conceptions of the self have had the capacity to be both oppressive and liberating, reinforcing imperial hierarchies through the pathologization of resistance to authority or subverting them in anti-colonial critique of the social pathology of colonialism and the cultural ignorance of Western-derived models for understanding non-Western psychologies (Anderson, Jenson and Keller, 2011). This comparative historical approach shares a number of concerns with the growing field of global history in its effort to engage in analyses of connections and comparisons across space, in its contributions to decentring historical narratives and in its emphasis on blurring conventional boundaries between peoples and places to focus on shared characteristics and experiences, mutual interdependence and relationships between the local, global and 'glocal' (Hopkins, 2002; Manning, 2003; Mazlish and Buultjens, 1993). I contend that efforts to develop histories of global mental health, and of global health more generally, should actively interrogate the relationship between these layered perspectives and, in so doing, integrate the history of global (mental) health with the practice of global history.

Nationalism, anti-colonialism and Nigerian psychiatry

In the Nigerian context the transformation of colonial psychiatry into a cross-cultural and global psychiatry was spearheaded mostly by indigenous Nigerian psychiatrists, trained in British or British-modelled universities and hospitals in the 1950s and 1960s, who took over mental health institutions as part of Nigerian decolonization and practised in the first few decades after independence in 1960. Initially, these psychiatrists had a nationalist agenda that promoted the dismantling of colonial knowledge and practices regarding mental health that had defined Africans as racial 'others' with inferior psyches to Europeans, and urged their replacement with indigenously inspired, culturally sensitive methods of research and practice. This nationalist agenda had a necessarily international, cross-cultural element to it, however. In order to deconstruct colonial knowledge systems that had defined Africans as mentally distinct from other racial groups, Nigerians not only had to conduct research within Nigeria to determine the nature of mental health and illness from a Nigerian perspective, but also to *compare* those results to other world populations. Nigerian psychiatrists therefore connected to, and in some cases created cross-cultural, transnational, efforts to determine the extent to which a universal understanding of the human psyche in its different cultural environments could be constructed and used to benefit the health and socio-economic development of a newly independent nation-state.

The best exemplar of this phase in Nigerian psychiatry was Thomas Adeoye Lambo (1923–2004). Lambo was Nigeria's first European-trained psychiatrist of indigenous background and the man who oversaw the transformation of Nigeria's psychiatric services in the 1950s from European-controlled institutions providing custodial care to a small number of extreme cases to Nigerian-controlled institutions providing diagnosis and treatment to the general population for the first time. Lambo was born and raised in Abeokuta, in south-west Nigeria. Educated in local mission schools, he travelled to the UK to undertake his medical training at the University of Birmingham in the 1940s (Sadowsky, 1997). Upon returning to Nigeria in 1951 he was briefly stationed at the Yaba Lunatic Asylum in Lagos. The experience, along with the encouragement of Dr Samuel Manuwa, who would become Nigeria's first indigenous director of medical services and, later, president of the World Federation for Mental Health, convinced him to make psychiatry his specialty (Asuni, 1967: 764). He then went back to the UK for further study at the Maudsley Hospital in London. The Maudsley was famous in psychiatric circles for its innovative approach. It shunned the notion of psychiatric hospital as custodial asylum, and instead focused heavily on treating voluntary psychoneurotic patients on an outpatient basis, a characteristic that greatly influenced Lambo's approach towards clinical practice (Jones, Rahaman and Woolven, 2007). When he returned to Nigeria Lambo immediately began to do things very differently than previous expatriate experts. Rather than work within the colonial-era construct that Western-styled psychiatric care was too expensive and culturally intrusive to work on African populations – which so many colonial officials had argued before him – Lambo went about actively trying to integrate 'modern' psychiatry with local cultural modalities. Indeed, Lambo's convictions about the importance of cultural sensitivity in psychiatric practice were so strong that he declared not Freud, Jung or Kraepelin, but the anthropologist Margaret Mead as the intellectual model for his pursuits (Sadowsky, 1999: 42 n.90). In emphasizing the importance of culture not only in presentation but also in treatment of mental illness, Lambo sought to transform psychiatry from a profession associated with ineffectuality and incarceration to one that Nigerians could associate with progress, national development and, most importantly, positive therapeutic results.

Much of Lambo's early work in this arena took place at Aro Mental Hospital, the first fully functioning mental hospital in Nigeria, which opened in 1954. The hospital was located just a couple of miles outside of Lambo's home town of Abeokuta, making Lambo particularly well suited for the task of developing strong relationships between the hospital and the surrounding communities. Rather than wait for the construction of the hospital to be completed (which did not happen until 1957), Lambo immediately began developing ways to provide psychiatric care outside the confines of the hospital walls. The result was the Aro Village Scheme, through which Lambo began to offer outpatient therapy in 1954. Based loosely on the famous community care schemes organized in Gheel, Belgium in the nineteenth century and, more recently, of Tigani al-Mahi in Sudan, the latter of which Lambo had toured personally,[2] the Aro Village Scheme provided a holistic, community-based therapeutic experience. Lambo made arrangements with local chiefs and elders for his patients to live in four villages surrounding Aro Hospital. Patients arrived with a family member – usually a mother, aunt or sister – who would keep watch over the patient during their stay. Patients attended the hospital during the day for regularly scheduled treatments which sometimes included such 'modern', up-to-date psychotherapeutic methods as electro-convulsion therapy, insulin-coma therapy and, by the late 1950s, psychopharmaceutical treatment, returning at night to the village, where they rented rooms in the homes of villagers. Patients and villagers engaged in community projects and activities together, including church services, films, plays, dances, and, eventually, in agricultural activities, which were meant to help patients develop qualities of sociability and responsibility that they would need for effective reintegration when they returned home (Asuni, 1967: 765).

Patients residing in the Aro village complex were admitted on a voluntary basis and could stay and receive treatment for as long as they liked. In practice, however, most stayed for less than three months. Factors determining length of stay were numerous. Some patients improved dramatically and went home. Others did not improve as much as was hoped, and family members decided to leave so as to seek alternative treatment. Still others left involuntarily, being unable to afford to stay longer, paying rent in the village while not working at home (Asuni, 1979: 41). Regardless, Lambo was able to declare that African patients treated within a culturally familiar community environment showed lower levels of chronicity and higher levels of permanent recovery than those treated in mental hospitals in Europe or the US, and at a lower cost than for prolonged inpatient care (Lambo, 1960a: 1697).[3]

While the hospital and the patients clearly benefited from association with the local villages, the villagers of Aro also had much to gain from their association with the hospital. Not only did the rents of patients and their relatives provide a steady source of income for villagers, but the hospital also became involved in the development planning of the village. Landlords could borrow money from the hospital to expand their operations and take in more patients (Park, 1960). The hospital helped to bring piped water, pit latrines and mosquito-eradication equipment to the village in the late 1950s (Lambo, 1960b: 198). Aro Hospital staff also provided medical treatment to villagers and their families (Asuni, 1967: 767).

With the village scheme up and running, the hospital itself continued to grow. It began admitting inpatients in 1957. Although it was originally designed to house 200 inpatients, with plans to increase to 500 beds over time, by the late 1960s only about 100 beds were in use at any given time, owing to staff constraints and a desire to maintain a focus on outpatient therapy. Despite the small number of inpatients served, by the late 1960s Aro boasted 'two admission wards, two infirmaries, three general treatment wards, and two disturbed wards' as well as a 'staff dining room, kitchen block, laundry, treatment block, student hostel, occupational therapy, main dining hall, administrative block, operating theater, gatekeeper's lodge and gate, and a number of both senior and junior residential buildings' (Asuni, 1967: 766).

Aro Hospital also became a major medical training centre. The hospital opened its own Psychiatric Nurses' School in 1956 and quickly became the centre of psychiatric nursing in the country, receiving nursing students from other Nigerian institutions, including the University of Ibadan, for rotations in the hospital and village by the mid-1960s (Asuni, 1967: 768). In 1979 Aro Neuropsychiatric Hospital, as it was by then known, became an official WHO Collaborating Centre for Research and Training, and in 1983 it added a Drug Addiction Research and Treatment Centre providing 24-hour service for substance abusers, the first facility of its kind in Nigeria (Makanjuola, 1986). It also established a department of psychology and began to provide postgraduate psychiatric training in conjunction with the West African College of Psychiatrists and a postgraduate programme in clinical psychology in conjunction with the University of Ibadan (Utomi, 1989: 691).

In 1963 Lambo left Aro Hospital to take up the position as Chair of the newly formed department of psychiatry at the University of Ibadan. He took the Aro Village Scheme with him (Asuni, 1967: 766). Daily rounds from nearby Aro Hospital were replaced with weekly rounds from the much more distant University Hospital, Ibadan, some forty miles away (Asuni, 1979: 39). Tolani Asuni, who had done his medical training in Dublin and arrived as an attendant physician at Aro in 1957, became the new director of Aro Mental Hospital, a position which he would hold until 1976. Asuni developed two new village schemes at Olomore and Idi-Ori, continuing Aro Hospital's dedication to the outpatient community care model (Asuni, 1967: 766).

Lambo's efforts to expand psychiatric service provision and tailor it to Nigerian needs and expectations should be seen not only in the context of a medical desire to provide effective care to individual patients but also as a contribution to the development and 'modernization' processes that Nigeria was undergoing alongside its political decolonization. Lambo, like colonial ethnopsychiatrists before him, believed that psychological maladjustment was on the increase in many African countries, including Nigeria, in the 1950s and 1960s. Although Lambo did not attribute this rise in maladjustment to any unique shortcomings of the 'African mind', as we will see below, he argued that the high levels of social disruption brought about by the widespread and rapid political, economic and social change affecting Nigerian society in the context of decolonization, development and 'modernization' schemes would be psychologically disruptive to human beings from any racial or cultural background. 'It is easier to see new buildings and new roads as evidence of progress,' declared Lambo, 'but unfortunately delinquency, prostitution, drug addiction and other social disasters accompanying "progress" are often tucked away from full view' (Lambo, 1965: 138). As rural–urban migration dislocated families and communities, and as values and lifestyles fluctuated to adjust to new possibilities and changing circumstances, Lambo believed that psychiatry had an important role to play in ushering Nigerians through this tumultuous time. He urged that the research agenda in the social sciences should be 'to investigate more scientific ways of preserving, activating, and mobilizing ... human resources for the balanced survival of our peoples and their optimal functioning in the new world' (Lambo, 1965: 134).

However, Lambo did not think it was sufficient for psychiatrists and social workers to shoulder the burden of the psychosocial fallout of Nigeria's development processes. He saw psychiatry as having a preventive medical component through its research and knowledge-gathering processes. If effective knowledge about the psychological effects of change on specific cultures could be produced, that information could then be transmitted to political leadership, which could in turn direct governmental policy toward an optimal balance between socioeconomic change and the public health needs of the population. In this way, he believed that 'psychiatry ... could contribute to national and individual productivity', (Lambo, 1982: 117) noting for example that schizophrenia tended to afflict young adults in the prime of their productive years. Finding a way to prevent psychotic breaks and to treat them effectively when they occurred had the potential to save Nigeria a great deal of cost in terms of long-term care as well as to prevent the wastage of manpower upon which development of the country relied. Lambo was himself active in integrating his psychiatric practice with the social and economic development of Nigeria. For example, at Aro Village he helped to organize occupational therapy programmes focused on farming. Patients receiving psychiatric care also therefore learned skills that would allow them to contribute productively to the survival of the village and to be productive members of society when they returned home (Asuni, 1967). In a speech to some of the young men engaged in these farming projects Lambo urged his patients to 'make a good success of what you are doing' so as to 'contribute to the economic and social life of Nigeria' (Park, 1960). For Lambo the psychological health of individual Nigerians was inextricably linked with the development of the country as a whole.

The actions that Lambo and other Nigerian psychiatrists took to develop 'modern' mental health services in Nigeria were not simply based in an agenda to import ideas from outside Africa, although this was certainly part of the story. However, the specific importations that he brought to Nigeria were ones that he felt would respond best to local circumstances and which would do the most to contribute to a nationalist, developmentalist agenda within the country. The motivations were largely internal. At the same time, the adaptations that Lambo made to his clinical processes through the Aro Village Scheme gained him international acclaim. Adaptations of the Aro village scheme were attempted in several other parts of Africa from the 1960s, including other parts of Nigeria, Senegal and Tanzania, among other places (Binitie, 1970; Bullard, 2005; Swift and Asuni, 1975: 215). In 1960 the UN filmed a documentary in Nigeria lauding the accomplishments of Lambo and his staff, called *The Healers of Aro* (Park, 1960). Lambo also later became highly involved in the development of international projects, serving as Deputy Director General of the WHO from 1973 to 1988, overseeing the development and implementation of projects not only in global mental health but in global health more generally. Local adaptations designed to meet nationalist, developmentalist interests therefore contributed to transformations in psychiatric practice in other parts of the world and resulted in the incorporation of Nigerian influences into the heart of international health structures.

Anti-colonialism, cultural nationalism and schizophrenia research

At Aro, Lambo also developed a research agenda that directly confronted the racist tenets of colonial psychiatry and sought to integrate African psychology into a universal model of human psychology on more equal terms through locally oriented studies on the nature of specific mental illnesses in Nigerian populations. These studies were at least partially motivated by anti-colonial and culturally nationalist sentiments prevalent in Nigeria and held by Lambo at the time. Lambo blasted generalizations of colonial psychiatrists who had argued for the intellectual and psychological inferiority of African peoples, declaring that existing research on mental disorder among Africans was 'extremely inadequate' because too often 'the clinical conclusions were founded on the treacherous sands of unscientific methodology' (Lambo, 1955:

241). He argued that colonial psychiatrists had hampered the practice of psychiatry in Africa, not by being actively ignorant of African cultures but 'by knowing so much that is not strictly true' (Lambo, 1955: 241). He parleyed his own cultural background as a Nigerian of Yoruba descent and his medical specialty in psychiatry from British universities to establish himself as a legitimate cross-cultural broker between the cultural particularities of African psyches and the universalist aspirations of psychiatric science.

One particular area in which Lambo was able to significantly critique established psychiatric knowledge about Africans was in the diagnosis of schizophrenia. As in other areas, he confronted significant racial baggage in the prevailing knowledge regarding schizophrenia in Africans in the 1950s. Colonial psychiatrists like the infamous J. C. Carothers of Mathari Hospital in Nairobi, Kenya, among others, defined Africans as innately more 'primitive' people than Europeans, and argued that, as such, Africans lived their everyday existences closer to the borderline between sanity and psychosis than Europeans did. For Carothers, 'the normal African is not schizophrenic, but the step from the primitive attitude to schizophrenia is but a short and easy one' (Carothers, 1940: 99). It is not surprising, then, that schizophrenia became by far the most common psychiatric diagnosis for African patients suffering from mental illness during the colonial era. In Kenya, Carothers identified over 28% of all patients as schizophrenic (Carothers, 1947: 570) and famously referred to schizophrenia as 'par excellence the chronic form of insanity in Africans as in Europeans' (Carothers, 1953: 139). The same held in Nigeria, where Cunyngham-Brown's 1938 survey of mental institutions revealed that roughly 20% of both asylum and home-care patients were classified as suffering from 'dementia praecox' (Cunyngham-Brown, 1938: 39).

As with other forms of mental illness, colonial psychiatrists were obsessed with the possibility that contact with European civilization, or 'detribalization', was somehow causing an increase in the prevalence of schizophrenia cases in African populations in the colonial context. The unproven theory suggested that the intrapersonal disruption brought about by the clash of 'primitive' and 'modern' worldviews created irreconcilable conflict within the African psyche, resulting in many cases in a psychotic break. As evidence, some colonial psychiatrists noted that the typical symptom complex associated with schizophrenia, particularly paranoia and delusions of grandeur, tended to occur in patients who had attained a significant degree of 'westernization', i.e. urbanization, European education, professional employment (Carothers, 1953: 140–142). However, some colonial psychiatrists also recognized that schizophrenia did, in fact, exist in rural communities relatively uncontaminated by European 'civilization'. Carothers noted that in rural Kenyans, for example, schizophrenia was 'common' and tended to manifest in delusions of persecution rather than the delusions of grandeur associated with classical Western schizophrenia (Carothers, 1953: 142).

When Lambo took the helm of Aro Mental Hospital he began almost immediately to engage what he saw as the deficiencies of colonial ethnopsychiatric research on schizophrenia in Africans and to insert Nigeria into the increasingly cross-cultural dialogue on the nature of schizophrenia. His earliest scientific publications were concerned primarily with the problem of diagnosing schizophrenia in Africans, and particularly with the role that culture played in shaping the symptomatology of schizophrenia (Lambo, 1955, 1957). In these articles Lambo addressed many of the assumptions of ethnopsychiatry and found them wanting. While he agreed with Western psychiatric models that posited schizophrenia as a cross-culturally universal phenomenon linked to brain biology, he vehemently objected to the idea that the culture of the 'normal' African exhibited psychotic tendencies that paved a short, easy path to a schizophrenic break. Reacting to the body of literature claiming that African beliefs in the mystical properties of things and of the omnipresence of supernatural forces represented the kind of 'logical' break characteristic of European schizophrenics, Lambo noted that 'primitive man's magic is no sign of a "pre-logical" mentality ... but of a "pre-causal" (that is, pre-scientific) thinking' (Lambo, 1955: 246). He noted that the ritual activities of African healers relied to a great extent on a consistent logic; it just happened not to conform to the scientific logic that European scientists trumpeted as the only objective form of 'reality' by which to judge sane behaviour. 'It would be a dangerous suggestion for scientific orientation to think that being different is being pathological,' he concluded (Lambo, 1955: 246).

Lambo also disagreed with the colonial psychiatric notion that rates of full-blown schizophrenia were probably lower among Africans in their indigenous cultures than among those 'detribalized' Africans struggling to 'modernize'. Whereas Carothers and others had argued that traditional, rural African cultures were relatively undemanding of individuals, allowing borderline and mild psychotic cases to pass undetected and even function more or less 'normally' (McCulloch, 1995: 52), Lambo believed that schizophrenic reactions were common in rural communities and that they reflected the 'psychic stresses which are inherent in the tribal culture' (Lambo, 1955: 240). He argued that one of the main reasons why colonial psychiatrists had assumed otherwise was because of their inability to identify schizophrenic symptoms when their cultural content differed from that found in Europeans.

In Lambo's own studies among his native Yoruba people he found that when significantly 'detribalized' Nigerians developed schizophrenia their symptoms tended to conform to those seen in people from a European cultural background. However, the symptoms of rural schizophrenics tended to differ from the classical European model. Lambo identified an 'atypical' set of symptoms more common in rural patients that included 'anxiety state, neurotic depression, vague hypochondriacal symptoms, magico-mystical projection symptoms, episodic twilight or confusional states, atypical depersonalisation phenomenon, emotional liability and retrospective falsification of hallucinatory experiences', representing a much broader symptom complex than that of the average European schizophrenic. A multiplicity of the atypical symptoms might be present in the rural non-literate patient at any given time, and they had a tendency to be transitory, according to Lambo. When delusions occurred, those of rural non-literate patients tended to exhibit content related to supernaturalism and ancestral cults, while literate, 'westernized' patients tended to express their delusions in the form of hypochondria more typical of Europeans (Lambo, 1955: 249–253).

However, despite the significant differences between the symptom complexes of the rural, non-literate and the classical forms of the disease, Lambo argued that this should not be seen as evidence of a 'peculiar native psychosis', since all the symptoms could be explained within existing psychodynamic formulations. He noted that 'aggressive excitement, restlessness and bizarre psychoneurotic features are not an uncommon accompaniment of all the principal forms of schizophrenia in any race or cultural group' (Lambo, 1957: 148), and that 'precipitating factors can be found if one looks for them in any environment' (Lambo, 1957: 150), indicating similarities where others might focus on difference. Indeed, the culturally specific features that Lambo emphasized existed 'only in addition to thought disorder, passivity feelings, affective disturbances, disturbed association of ideas and other symptoms', which Lambo found to be 'varying aspects of the fundamental schizophrenic order common to both [literate, urban and non-literate, rural] groups' (Lambo, 1955: 253).

The overall picture for Lambo was one in which schizophrenia was a universal disorder the content of which was determined by cultural markers. In this way the African psyche, regardless of its cultural background, functioned no differently than that of any other human being whose reactions to stimuli were also culturally determined but not necessarily culturally caused. For Lambo, the fact that the manifestation of schizophrenia looked different in urban, literate and rural, non-literate Nigerians was proof of the fact that the 'innate psychological qualities' of Europeans and Africans did not actually differ substantially. If they did, it should be expected that westernized Yoruba men would react differently to the stresses of modern civilization than Europeans because of differences in constitutional factors. That those Nigerians most acculturated to European ways exhibited similar form and content of schizophrenia to Europeans indicated that they assimilated cultural cues in much the same way that Europeans did and were therefore psychologically similar to Europeans, despite their racial difference. Lambo believed that his findings went a long way towards disproving some of the more outrageously racist claims of colonial psychiatrists and declared that 'on the basis of deeper psychological determinants, this investigation has shown that the aphorism "the nature of men is identical; what divides them is their custom," is a valid statement even at the level of psychotic regression' (Lambo, 1955: 242).

After a few years of using his new diagnostic criteria for schizophrenia in clinical practice Lambo provided data from Aro Hospital indicating the significant levels of rural schizophrenia that had been uncovered through greater engagement with rural communities. By 1960, of 960 schizophrenic patients treated at Aro Hospital, only 370 were urban and literate, while 270 were rural, the remaining quotient being urban and illiterate. These numbers masked the reality that large numbers of rural schizophrenics were still not seeking treatment at psychiatric hospitals (Lambo, 1960a: 1696).

While Lambo was adamant that the cultural impact on schizophrenia in Africans was not an indication of differences in causality, he became increasingly interested in the possibility that cultural factors might have a significant effect on the prognosis of individual schizophrenic patients. By the early 1960s Lambo had become aware that 'lack of complete regression and of severe chronicity' was 'remarkably noticeable in African schizophrenics' as compared to European patients. Of the 960 schizophrenic patients treated at Aro Hospital between 1954 and 1959 Lambo noted that 486 had improved to the point that they could go home and resume some, possibly all, of their normal responsibilities in their communities (Lambo, 1960a: 1696). This was a remission rate of over 50% for Nigerian patients at a time when most Euro-American studies showed improvement rates of 20–40% (WHO, 1979: 20–23). Lambo further noted that 'permanent recovery ... seems to occur much more readily in African patients, probably more often than has been generally supposed by experienced workers in Western culture' (Lambo, 1960a: 1697). He attributed the lack of chronicity in African patients partly to 'genetic and constitutional factors', but believed that environmental and cultural factors played a key role in this outcome. 'Assuming that genetic endowment, especially in respect of predisposition to schizophrenia, is similar in all ethnic groups', he hypothesized that 'the difference in the course and outcome of the disorders can only be found in the differential cultural conditioning to which these people have been subjected' (Lambo, 1960a: 1697). Lambo credited the cultural emphasis on community care in African healing systems, and his own reformulation of it at Aro Village, as the most apparent contributor to the recovery and reintegration of African schizophrenics into their societies, and suggested that prolonged institutionalization in Western hospital settings might actually exacerbate chronicity in European and American patients.

Cross-cultural psychiatry and the international pilot study of schizophrenia

Lambo was not the first or only Western-trained psychiatrist to suggest that schizophrenia looked different in different cultures. Indeed, the type of work that Lambo was doing fitted naturally into a growing network of cross-cultural psychiatry that was beginning to compile and share data on schizophrenia from across the world. In the 1950s and 1960s a number of studies of schizophrenia from a variety of different cultural settings illustrated that although Western-trained psychiatrists were diagnosing schizophrenia in all racial, cultural and social groups, the typical form and content of schizophrenia looked different in different places. For example, beginning in the late 1950s, the group of cross-cultural psychiatrists at McGill University in Montreal began trying to compile and synthesize data on schizophrenia diagnosis in various parts of the world. Using the network developed through the distribution of the *Transcultural Psychiatric Review and Newsletter*, E. D. Wittkower, H. B. M. Murphy, J. Fried and H. Ellenberger sent out questionnaires to psychiatrists working in different cultural environments to learn what their field experience taught them about schizophrenia in their respective territories. Respondents returned thirty-seven questionnaires from twenty-five different countries encompassing the six inhabited continents, including data from Nigeria.

By the early 1960s the WHO had also begun the process of systematizing the compilation of epidemiological data on schizophrenia around the world. In 1959 the WHO declared an interest in promoting cross-cultural psychiatric epidemiology, and spent the next several years developing an effective methodology for a broad-based study. The result was the International Pilot Study of Schizophrenia (IPSS), launched in 1966 to test whether effective criteria for diagnosing schizophrenia cross-culturally could be determined. Nine centres across the globe were designated as catchment areas for the accumulation of data. Ibadan, Nigeria was one of them.[4] From 1966 to 1971 Lambo served as the chief collaborating investigator of the Ibadan group. Tolani Asuni also served as a collaborating investigator during this period before taking over as chief collaborating investigator for the period 1971–76. The Nigerian catchment area accounted for a plurality of all the patients included in the data analysis, providing 145 of the 1,202 cases analysed, slightly more than one-ninth of the study group (WHO, 1973: 161).

The findings of cross-cultural research into schizophrenia around the world tended to confirm the conclusions that Lambo had reached based on Nigerian circumstances. Studies conducted in Europe and Asia in the 1950s supported his contention that rural schizophrenia was not uncommon. Asian studies also found, similarly to Lambo, that the form of schizophrenia among non-westernized individuals tended to follow the pattern of aggression, excitement and confusional state, following a course of acute onset but relatively benign long-term prognosis (WHO, 1973: 25–30). Cross-cultural studies also found, in concordance with Lambo, that symptom content varied culturally. The results of the McGill study in 1960 indicated that, at a broad level, psychiatrists the world over did agree on what the typical characteristics of schizophrenia were: namely, 'social and emotional withdrawal, hallucinations and delusions, and flatness of affect' (Wittkower, Murphy, Fried and Ellenberger, 1960: 855). However, beyond this basic agreement results diverged significantly on the frequency of subtypes and symptom content. According to the responses, paranoid schizophrenia was common everywhere, but other subtypes of schizophrenia varied significantly across space. For example, catatonic schizophrenia was much more common among Japanese and Indian patients than Euro-American ones. Furthermore, the content of specific symptoms varied greatly as well. While auditory hallucinations were generally common, visual hallucinations were much more common in African and Middle Eastern patients than in other groups. Where delusions were common, their content was much more likely to be religious in nature in Christian and Muslim groups than in others. Japanese and Indian patients were characterized as experiencing flatness of affect more frequently than other groups (Murphy, Wittkower, Fried and Ellenberger, 1963: 247). In fact, in fifteen cultures, flatness of affect was categorized as an infrequent symptom, despite its being universally recognized as a basic characteristic of the disease.

Similarly, the IPSS noted in the publication of its first volume of results in 1973 that all nine catchment areas were able to consistently differentiate schizophrenia from major affective disorders, although there were some anomalies. For example, it was found, famously, that the American and Soviet definitions of what qualified as schizophrenia were significantly broader than those adhered to by the other seven research centres (WHO, 1973: 168–175). However, perhaps the most important finding of the WHO project came from a follow-up study conducted two years later. In the follow-up study investigators tracked down patients from the original study to see how they were managing their illness. The results indicated that patients from non-Western backgrounds had a much more favourable long-term prognosis than those of from Europe and the US (WHO, 1979: 113–164). Of all the groups, the Ibadan patients had the best outcomes, with 46% reporting full remission. 97% had stayed out of hospital for at least three-quarters of the time since the initial study (WHO, 1979: 163). The findings of the follow-up study therefore confirmed the impressions that Lambo had noted twenty years earlier: that African schizophrenics were much less likely to develop chronicity than Euro-Americans.

These cross-cultural studies ultimately raised more questions than they answered. Methodological complications and logistical issues allowed for significant criticism of the findings and little agreement on what the results meant. Clearly, psychiatrists the world over agreed that something called schizophrenia in the Western definitional sense *did* exist universally in human cultures, but there were clearly some significant differences in the ways that psychiatrists around the world were diagnosing it. However, what the cross-cultural syntheses of the 1960s and 1970s could not prove was whether these differences resulted from differences in the diagnostic judgements of individual psychiatrists or whether they actually arose from differences in the ways that cultural factors influenced the course of schizophrenia. It was not at all clear where the boundaries of any given culture should be set. Although responses came from twenty-five different countries in the McGill study, and nine different countries in the IPSS, the religious, ethnic, social and cultural backgrounds were undoubtedly very diverse within and across these national boundaries. Psychiatrists themselves often did not share a cultural background with their patients, making issues of communication and bias more problematic in the diagnostic process. Ultimately, Wittkower and colleagues concluded that their 1960 findings indicated 'a major barrier for transcultural comparison' (Wittkower et al., 1960: 862). Cross-cultural psychiatrists also criticized the process of the IPSS, noting that it paid far more attention to social indicators (e.g. marital status, education level, wealth etc.) than to explicitly cultural factors in its analysis. Others criticized the incomprehensiveness of the IPSS findings (it was, after all, only a pilot study) and its inability to provide a perfectly acceptable and encompassing definition of schizophrenia for universal application (Edgerton, 1980: 167–189; Murphy, 1986: 19).

Criticisms aside, transcultural psychiatric research on schizophrenia clearly provided an outlet and an opportunity for Lambo to achieve a broader agenda of reforming racialized conceptions of mental illness developed under colonial power structures. Presenting schizophrenia as a universal mental illness masked by pathoplastic cultural overlay promoted his cultural politics of equality. Cross-cultural evidence that cultural variation of schizophrenic form and content was universal promoted the concept of the innate equality of human psychological function. Data demonstrating that non-westerners recovered more readily from schizophrenia suggested that Western psychiatry had something to learn from non-Western cultures and healing regimes. Lambo's personal research suggested these conclusions at a local level in the 1950s; international networks of transcultural psychiatric research reinforced them at a global level in the 1960s and 1970s. The process of the IPSS was not simply a story of external force acting upon Africans but, rather, was itself partly shaped by Lambo's personal cultural politics that developed out of decades of experience as a Yoruba Nigerian, a colonial subject and an anti-colonial nationalist in a time of great social transformations in his country. And Ibadan was only one of nine research centres in the study, all of which were steeped in their own local and national contexts. The contours of global schizophrenia research were shaped by the convergence of a variety of different local, national and regional interests that all had a stake in the outcomes of cross-cultural psychiatric research.

Conclusion

The history of the development of mental health research and services in Nigeria complicates notions of the global that rely on a narrative of external, Western-based motivation, resources and agendas by illustrating not only how health professionals have reshaped those external influences to meet local and national concerns but also how those localizations contribute to the shaping of the global itself. This type of circulation of ideas within networks of scholars and practitioners is not a revelation: historians have increasingly utilized it to explain circuits of scientific knowledge production and dissemination over several centuries within European empires (Lester, 2006; Raj, 2007). At the same time, the notion that African health systems are historically dynamic and pluralistic is equally well established (Feierman, 1985; Janzen, 1978). If we are going to make claims that contemporary processes and structures of global health have historical antecedents in the colonial and post-war international health eras, which they clearly do in many ways, then we also need to come to terms with the complexity of interactions that characterized those previous regimes of knowledge production, dissemination and application so as to better articulate the nature of the relationship between the past and the present.

Most notably for present purposes, this coming to terms requires a reconceptualization of how humanistic scholarship represents peoples and cultures and the effects that they have on each other. Binary relics of colonial and post-colonial analysis are too easily reproduced in reverse engineering a history of global health in Africa. The tendency to see the 'global' as a set of forces outside of and separate from 'Africa', rather than as a set of forces that have been created in part through incorporation of African people, resources and knowledge, reinforces a spatial (and to a certain extent racial) colonizer/colonized dichotomy that social and cultural historians have been blurring for several decades (Cooper, 2005). Such recognition does not deflect the critiques that have been levelled at international and global health structures and institutions in the post-colonial context, particularly those related to psychiatry and mental health, but it does potentially reshape how we think about the content, capacity and boundaries of their hegemony. In so doing, it is my hope that we can begin do develop a more explicitly global history of global health and global mental health in Africa and beyond.

Notes

1 The body of this chapter was originally published in my historical monograph *Black Skin, White Coats: Nigerian Psychiatrists, Decolonization, and the Globalization of Psychiatry*. I would like to thank Ohio University Press for permission to reproduce it here.
2 As noted by al-Mahi in his introductory comments at the First Pan-African Psychiatric Conference (Lambo, 1961: 11).
3 Although he gives no figures.
4 The others were Aarhus, Denmark; Agra, India; Cali, Colombia; London; Moscow; Taipei; Prague; and Washington, DC.

References

Anderson, Warwick, Deborah Jenson and Richard C. Keller (eds) (2011) *Unconscious Dominions: Psychoanalysis, Colonial Trauma, and Global Sovereignties*. Durham, NC: Duke University Press.

Asuni, Tolani (1967) 'Aro Hospital in Perspective', *American Journal of Psychiatry* 124 (6), 763–770.
Asuni, Tolani (1979) 'Therapeutic Communities of the Hospital and Villages in Aro Hospital Complex in Nigeria', *African Journal of Psychiatry* 1, 35–42.
Bell, Leland V. (1991) *Mental and Social Disorder in Sub-Saharan Africa: The Case of Sierra Leone, 1787–1990*. Westport, CT: Greenwood Press.
Binitie, Ayo (1970) 'Experiences in the Development of Psychiatric Services in Mid-Western State of Nigeria', *Psychopathologie africaine* 6, 201–208.
Bullard, Alice (2005) 'The Critical Impact of Frantz Fanon and Henri Collomb: Race, Gender and Personality Testing of North and West Africans', *Journal of the History of Behavioral Sciences* 41 (3), 225–248.
Carothers, J. C. (1940) 'Some Speculations on Insanity in Africans in General', *East African Medical Journal* 17, 90–105.
Carothers, J. C. (1947) 'A Study of Mental Derangement in Africans, and an Attempt to Explain Its Peculiarities, More Especially in Relation to the African Attitude to Life', *Journal of Mental Science* 93, 548–597.
Carothers, J. C. (1953) *The African Mind in Health and Disease: A Study in Ethnopsychiatry*. Geneva: World Health Organization.
Cooper, Frederic (2005) *Colonialism in Question: Theory, Knowledge, History*. Berkeley: University of California Press.
Cunyngham-Brown, Robert (1938) *Report III on the Care and Treatment of the Mentally Ill in British West African Colonies*. London: Garden City Press.
Deacon, Harriet Jane (1996) 'Madness, Race and Moral Treatment: Robben Island Lunatic Asylum, Cape Colony, 1846–1890', *History of Psychiatry* vii, 287–297.
Edgerton, Robert B. (1980) 'Traditional Treatment for Mental Illness in Africa: A Review', *Culture, Medicine and Psychaitry* 4, 167–89.
Fanon, Frantz (1967) *Black Skin, White Masks*. Translated by Charles Lam Markmann. New York: Grove Press. First published 1952.
Fanon, Frantz (1978) *The Wretched of the Earth*. Translated by Constance Farrington. New York: Monthly Review Press. First published 1961.
Feierman, Steven (1985) 'Struggles for Control: The Social Roots of Health and Healing in Modern Africa', *African Studies Review* 28 (2–3), 73–147.
Hodge, Joseph Morgan (2007) *Triumph of the Expert: Agrarian Doctrines of Development and the Legacies of British Colonialism*. Athens, OH: Ohio University Press.
Hopkins, A. G. (2002) 'The History of Globalization – and the Globalization of History?', in *Globalization in World History*, edited by A. G. Hopkins, 1–44. New York and London: W. W. Norton and Company.
Jackson, Lynette (2005) *Surfacing Up: Psychiatry and Social Order in Colonial Zimbabwe, 1908–1968*. Ithaca, NY: Cornell University Press.

Janzen, John M. (1978) *The Quest for Therapy in Lower Zaire.* Berkeley: University of California Press.
Jones, Edgar, Shahina Rahaman and Robin Woolven (2007) 'The Maudsley Hospital: Design and Strategic Direction, 1923-39', *Medical History* 51 (3), 357-378.
Keller, Richard C. (2007) *Colonial Madness: Psychiatry in French North Africa.* Chicago: University of Chicago Press.
Lambo, T. Adeoye (1955) 'The Role of Cultural Factors in Paranoid Psychosis among the Yoruba Tribe', *Journal of Mental Science* 101, 239-266.
Lambo, T. Adeoye (1957) 'Some Unusual Features of Schizophrenia among Primitive Peoples', *West African Medical Journal* 6, 147-152.
Lambo, T. Adeoye (1960a) 'Further Neuropsychiatric Observations in Nigeria', *British Medical Journal* 2 (1060), 1696-1704.
Lambo, T. Adeoye (1960b) 'A Form of Social Psychiatry in Africa', *World Mental Health* 13, 190-203.
Lambo, T. Adeoye (ed.) (1961) *First Pan-African Psychiatric Conference, Abeokuta,Nigeria.* Ibadan: Government Printer.
Lambo, T. Adeoye (1965) 'Socioeconomic Changes in Africa and Their Implications for Mental Health', in *Man in Africa,* ed. Gordon Wolstenholme and Maeve O'Connor (pp. 121-45). Boston: Little, Brown.
Lambo, T. Adeoye (1982) 'Thomas Lambo', in *Psychiatrists on Psychiatry,* ed. Michael Shepherd (pp. 98-123). Cambridge: Cambridge University Press.
Langwick, Stacey, Hansjörg Dilger and Abdoulaye Kane (2012) 'Introduction: Transnational Medicine, Mobile Experts', in *Medicine, Mobility, and Power in Global Africa,* ed. Hansjörg Dilger, Abdoulaye Kane and Stacey Langwick (pp. 1-27). Bloomington: Indiana University Press.
Lester, Alan (2006) 'Imperial Circuits and Networks: Geographies of the British Empire', *History Compass* 4 (1), 124-141.
Makanjuola, J. D. A. (1986) 'The Aro Drug Addiction Research and Treatment Centre: A First Report', *British Journal of Addiction* 81, 809-14.
Manning, Patrick (2003) *Navigating World History: Historians Create a Global Past.* New York: Palgrave Macmillan.
Mazlish, Bruce and Ralph Buultjens (eds) (1993) *Conceptualizing Global History.* Boulder, CO: Westview Press.
McCulloch, Jock (1995) *Colonial Psychiatry and 'the African Mind'.* Cambridge: Cambridge University Press.
Murphy, H. B. M. (1986) 'Historical Development of Transcultural Psychiatry', in *Transcultural Psychiatry,* ed. John L. Cox (pp. 7-22). London: Croom Helm.
Murphy, H. B. M., E. D. Wittkower, J. Fried and H. Ellenberger (1963) 'A Crossculturual Survey of Schizophrenic Symptomatology', *International Journal of Social Psychiatry* 9, 237-249.

Park, Ben (1960) Film. *The Healers of Aro*. New York: United Nations.
Prince, Ruth J. (2013) 'Introduction: Situating Health and the Public in Africa', in *Making and Unmaking Public Health in Africa: Ethnographic and Historical Perspectives*, ed. Ruth J. Prince and Rebecca Marsland (pp. 1–51). Athens: Ohio University Press.
Raj, Kapil (2007) *Relocating Modern Science: Circulation and the Construction of Knowledge in South Asia and Europe, 1650–1900*. New York: Palgrave Macmillan.
Sadowsky, Jonathan (1997) 'Thomas Adeoye Lambo', in *Doctors, Nurses, and Medical Practitioners: A Bio-Bibliographical Sourcebook*, ed. Lois N. Magner (pp. 172–176). Westport, CT: Greenwood Press.
Sadowsky, Jonathan (1999) *Imperial Bedlam: Institutions of Madness in Colonial Southwest Nigeria*. Berkeley: University of California Press.
Swift, Charles R. and Tolani Asuni (1975) *Mental Health and Disease in Africa: With Special Reference to Africa South of the Sahara*. New York: Churchill Livingstone.
Tilley, Helen (2011) *Africa as a Living Laboratory: Empire, Development, and the Problem of Scientific Knowledge, 1870–1950*. Chicago: University of Chicago Press.
Utomi, D. O. (1989) 'Clinical Psychology at Aro Psychiatric Hospital', in *Clinical Psychology in Africa (South of the Sahara, the Caribbean and Afro-Latin America)*, ed. Karl Peltzer and Peter O. Ebigbo (pp. 691–695). Enugu: Working Group for African Psychology.
Vaughan, Megan (1983) 'Idioms of Madness: Zomba Lunatic Asylum, Nyasaland, in the Colonial Period', *Journal of Southern African Studies* 9 (2), 218–238.
Webb, James L. A. and Tamara Giles-Vernick (2013) 'Introduction', in *Global Health in Africa: Historical Perspectives on Disease Control*, ed. Tamara Giles-Vernick and James L. A. Webb, Jr (pp. 1–21). Athens: Ohio University Press.
Wittkower, E. D., H. B. Murphy, J. Fried and H. Ellenberger (1960) 'Crosscultural Inquiry into the Symptomatology of Schizophrenia', *Annals of the New York Academy of Science* 84, 854–863.
WHO (1973) *International Pilot Study on Schizophrenia*. Geneva: World Health Organization.
WHO (1979) *Schizophrenia: An International Follow-up Study*. Geneva: World Health Organization.

5

'Clearing the streets': enacting human rights in mental health care in Ghana

Ursula M. Read

Clearing the streets

In 2014 Dr Osei, the leader of the newly established Mental Health Authority in Ghana, launched a programme named Operation Clear the Streets. He described the operation, publicized in the local media, as a response to 'numerous concerns expressed by the general public about the patients roaming the streets of Accra and other cities and towns'. Although Dr Osei acknowledged that similar operations had taken place during large events attended by international visitors, such as the celebration of the fiftieth anniversary of Ghana's independence in 2007, he went to some lengths to distinguish the programme from earlier efforts to rid the capital's streets of unsightly vagrants. This was a targeted programme rather than an indiscriminate clean-up: 'if we bring a lot it is like we are bringing rubbish from the streets, but they are human beings'. This time the aim was to 'repatriate' the vagrants to their communities, rather than simply round them up and confine them in the psychiatric hospital, where they would add to the chronic overcrowding and, importantly, the burden on the public purse. He explained that the programme was explicitly designed to promote the rehabilitation of those apprehended by admitting them to the hospital for treatment: 'We bring them in, clean them up, treat them, treat any physical health problems, when they are well enough we integrate them into the community, link them up with their families.' The ultimate aim was, he said, 'a situation where in five years' time there will be no mentally ill roaming the street'.

Despite this reframing of the operation as a process of treatment and rehabilitation, rather than confinement, the operation provoked a backlash from Human Rights Watch (HRW) and other international agencies. HRW declared that enforcing the involuntary treatment of homeless persons was a breach of their human rights. However, Dr Osei robustly defended the operation by remarking that he was merely fulfilling the mandate of Ghana's Mental Health Act, which had been passed two years previously. A media report quoted him citing from the Act: 'The Mental Health Act 846 of 2012, Section 73, and Subsection 1–7 on "Mentally ill found in public places" allows us, in fact, mandates us to take these patients to "a place of safety" and treatment, on Certificate of Urgency.' According to the news report, he compared the operation to the 'sectioning' of patients under the British Mental Health Act, claiming that as a result 'mental patients were not found on the streets of London, except destitute or homeless'. He added: 'Insistence that a vagrant psychotic, who lives in his own world, should give informed consent is standing logic on its head and does not show enough appreciation of the nature of mental illness.'[1]

The discourse of human rights has a long genealogy in relation to the treatment of persons with mental illness and has become a central narrative in the transnational networks and activities which have come to be characterized as global mental health. Indeed, appeals to the human rights of persons with mental illness have formed a moral argument for intervention to improve mental health care worldwide (Patel, Saraceno and Kleinman, 2006). The reform of mental health law in Ghana would seem to be of a piece with the progressive vision of global mental health, in which internationally agreed standards inform the development of humane mental health services. Indeed, proposals for Ghana's new Mental Health Act became a flagship example for WHO's programme on mental health law reform (WHO, 2007) and the Act has been hailed as a 'success story' in the region (Alem and Manning, 2016: 312). Nonetheless, as this scenario demonstrates, the implementation of the new legislation has proved less than straightforward. This could be read as an example of 'culture clash' between a global vision of human rights and local interpretation. Sally Engel Merry outlines the challenges for 'human rights translators' such as Dr Osei, who must appeal to both international donors and local communities in enacting rights-based policies. Nonetheless, rather than illustrating a clash between two 'culturally distinct social worlds' (Merry, 2006: 38), what is striking in this scenario is the ways in which it interweaves colonial and post-colonial genealogies and dispositions, while engaging with unresolved ethical and social questions regarding the use of coercion in psychiatry (Molodynski, Rugkasa and Burns, 2016). The colonial terminology of 'vagrant psychotics' and public concerns about the wandering mad thus sit alongside comparison of UK and Ghanaian mental health law and psychiatry's claims to professional expertise regarding the decision-making capacity of persons with mental illness. In this respect the scenario illustrates less a contrast between an explicitly global articulation of human rights, as exemplified by HRW, WHO and the UN, and local concerns regarding vagrant madmen than a 'global assemblage' (Collier and Ong, 2005). In Collier and Ong's conceptualization the 'global assemblage' is the interaction of global forms, such as human rights, with other elements 'occupying a common field in contingent, uneasy, unstable interrelationships' (Collier and Ong, 2005: 12). The frictions arising within such 'zones of awkward engagement' are precisely what stimulate the movement and action of global forms (Tsing, 2005), making them meaningful in novel ways.

Seeing human rights and mental health care in Ghana as a global assemblage perturbs the temporal trajectory of psychiatric reform from institutionalization to community care. Several scholars describe the discomforting 'ghostly presences' which haunt modernization projects in post-colonial psychiatry (Kilroy-Marac, 2019; Street, 2018; Varley and Varma, 2018). Describing the neglect of persons with chronic mental illness within India's moves to community mental health care, Varley and Varma reveal 'the incompleteness of global and national projects enacting modern, scientific, and humane psychiatry' (Varley and Varma, 2018: 640). These chronic patients, like the 'vagrant psychotics', are jinn or ghosts, the haunting presence of the asylum past and 'matter out of place' within the partially realized reform of India's mental health service (Varma, 2016). However, in Alice Street's formulation (Street, 2018) such hauntings are also ethical critique – iatrogenic harms are the 'ghostly presence' within biomedical practices, challenging progressive narratives of humane reform. Ghana's Mental Health Act is haunted not just by colonial histories of social cleansing and control of wandering 'lunatics', but by psychiatry's own iatrogenic potentiality and the enduring power hierarchies which mark relationships between the global

North and South. In her investigation of the legacy of the Fann clinic in Dakar, Senegal, Katie Kilroy-Marac cites Achille Mbembe on the particular 'entanglements' of the post-colony – 'an overlapping of different, intersected and entwined threads in tension with one another' (Kilroy-Marac, 2019: 25). As this scenario makes clear, as the head of psychiatry in Ghana, Dr Osei is caught up in such entanglements and tensions between national and international institutions. An indispensable collaborator in global mental health programmes in the country, through his frequent media appearances Dr Osei has also become the public face of mental health in Ghana, attempting to educate the populace on the scientific and humanitarian claims of psychiatry and the necessity to implement the Mental Health Act. In his performance as both global actor and local broker (Yarrow, 2011) Dr Osei draws on a 'moral and ethical assemblage' of institutional, public and personal discourses (Zigon, 2010) to articulate a position which resonates both with international psychiatric practice and human rights and with local expectations of his role. However, even within these two spheres there are potential conflicts or contradictions between different actors, such as between mental health service user organizations and psychiatrists, or between policy makers and the general public.

This chapter describes the various historical and contemporary traces entangled in this particular 'ethical moment' (Zigon, 2010) in the articulation of global mental health in the context of Ghana. First, I describe the ways in which, since the 1990s, human rights have emerged as a dominant narrative in what has become global mental health, while obscuring the controversies and dilemmas which continue to trouble the practice of mental health care worldwide – notably the involuntary treatment of persons believed to be suffering from mental illness and the historical tensions between psychiatry's role in providing medical care and controlling social deviance (Brodwin and Velpry, 2014). Second, I trace the history of psychiatry in Ghana from the colonial period to the era of global mental health to show how Operation Clear the Streets reframes historic concerns regarding the 'vagrant psychotic' (Baasher et al., 1983) within a discourse of 'community integration' as well as legitimized coercive practices in contemporary mental health practice. For Osei, as for colonial and postcolonial authorities (de-Graft Aikins, 2015), clearing the streets is part and parcel of Ghana's progress towards modern statehood, in which the presence of dishevelled and dirty homeless persons in urban spaces is a sign of incomplete development. Despite the promotion of legislative reform as protecting the human rights of persons with mental illness, as with Operation Clear the Streets, mental health legislation retains its coercive power, particularly where investment in health and support services is lacking (Lund et al., 2012). At the same time a therapeutic rationale for such coercion enables Dr Osei to speak to a globalized humanitarian ethos of deinstitutionalization and community care in keeping with the accepted standards of 'a modern mental health service' (Thornicroft and Tansella, 2004).[2]

Global mental health and human rights

Concerns around human rights have a long genealogy in psychiatry, producing defining moments in the discipline's foundational mythology. From the unchaining of patients by Pinel at the end of the eighteenth century (Keller, 2005), to the closing of psychiatric hospitals pioneered by Franco Basaglia in the 1960s (Scheper-Hughes and Lovell, 1986), the language of rights revolved largely around freedom from the horrors of the asylum and confinement, coercion and restraint. The history of psychiatry over the period was of course something less than a simple trajectory from brutality to enlightenment, and processes of what came to be called 'psychiatric reform' were unevenly realized. Coercion and confinement of various kinds remain a central tool of mental health care in most jurisdictions, even as asylums have closed and community mental health care has expanded (Molodynski, Rugkasa and Burns, 2016; Saya et al., 2019). Indeed, practices of confinement have arguably been reconfigured from 'old' to 'new' institutions, most notoriously from asylums to prisons (Gostin, 2008; Lovell and Rhodes, 2014). Nonetheless, the application of human rights to mental health paralleled in many ways the wider promotion of a universal humanitarianism, from the rights of man to the founding constitutions of the UN and WHO. In the 1960s opposition to compulsory psychiatric detention and treatment in the US took inspiration from the civil rights movement, with people who had experienced involuntary confinement coming together to advocate for their rights. Some successfully launched appeals against their commitment, and a 1966 court ruling established the principle of the 'least restrictive' alternative for treatment of psychiatric conditions (Testa and West, 2010). Although Italy pioneered the move from institutional to community-based care, policies of 'deinstitutionalization' were adopted in the US in the 1960s, followed by the UK and other European states from the 1970s (Fakhoury and Priebe, 2002; Thornicroft and Bebbington, 1989). However, in the late 1980s a media exposé of the appalling conditions in the psychiatric hospital on the Greek island of Leros highlighted the enduring injustices faced by persons with mental illness in state-sponsored institutions (Giannakopoulos and Anagnostopoulos, 2016). This led to a UN inquiry and the publication of the UN Principles for the Protection of Persons with Mental Illness and the Improvement of Mental Health Care, otherwise known as the MI Principles (United Nations, 1991). The emphasis on protection and care reflects a dual orientation towards the reduction of coercive treatment under the principle of 'the least restrictive environment' and the provision of community-based services as central to humane mental health care.

The publication of *World Mental Health: Problems and Priorities in Developing Countries* by a prominent group of anthropologists and psychiatrists at Harvard University (Desjarlais et al., 1995) also focused attention on abuses in psychiatric institutions. As evidenced in the title, this time the scope of comparison embraced countries from Latin America to Asia, prefiguring the global scale on which mental health (as with global health) was coming to be envisaged. Stigma, neglect and abuse, as well as the lack of mental health services, particularly community-based mental health care, were emphasized throughout the volume. *World Mental Health* was the first publication on mental health to cite the World Bank GBD statistics, which brought new visibility to mental disorders as contributors to disability and premature mortality and enabled comparison across countries. The WHO World Health Report of 2001, *Mental Health: New Understanding, New Hope* (WHO 2001), also cited the GBD to make a moral case for treatment and promoted the provision of mental health services within primary care rather than specialized institutions as a means to protect the human rights of persons with mental illness.

The 2001 Report could be viewed as the founding artefact of global mental health, since when an expanding network of academics, clinicians, NGOs and patient advocates, otherwise known as 'service users', have pushed for greater international attention to mental health. From the outset the language of human rights has been central to the rhetoric of global mental health (Cooper, 2015), defining an imperative for action to address what is presented as an urgent humanitarian crisis of unmet need. This has been depicted by WHO and others as a 'treatment gap' between those made visible via the GBD metrics as in need of treatment and the resources available to treat them (Kohn et al., 2004). In 2007 an influential series of articles published in *The Lancet* argued forcefully for the 'scaling up' of interventions to reduce the burden of mental illness (Lancet Global Mental Health Group, 2007). In this argument treatment and care was presented as a right denied to the poorest and most vulnerable populations of the world.

The same year in which the World Health Report was published a fire at a shrine in Erwardi, India led to the deaths of several people being treated for mental illness who were chained to stakes and unable to escape (Murthy, 2001). Like Leros, this brought international attention, this time focused on human rights abuses within traditional healing centres rather than hospitals. Such a picture presented a challenge to earlier depictions of traditional healers as benign alternatives to psychiatry, in which the use of mechanical restraints evoked little concern. Harding, for example, who studied the operations of a traditional healer in Nigeria in the 1970s, stated that while many 'Western psychiatrists' objected to the use of mechanical restraint and confinement by traditional healers, their use was mitigated in the long term by the 'concern and care' shown by the healer towards his patients (Harding, 1973). Since Erwardi a number of reports have depicted the use of chains and other forms of restraint on persons with mental illness across the globe, including in Ghana, as well as exposing the continuing failures of psychiatric institutions. An article in *Nature* in 2011 by a consortium of influential figures in global mental health identified 'grand challenges' for mental health research, including ways to reduce stigma and social exclusion and to improve access to 'evidence-based' care (Collins et al., 2011). The article was accompanied by two photographs which reflected these twin spheres of concern: in one a young Somali girl sits in chains on the bare ground, in another a group of women stand disconsolately in a bare room in a Ukrainian psychiatric hospital.

Following the publication of the World Health Report the WHO Mental Health Division began to promote legislative reform as a central tool in protecting the human rights of persons with mental disorder. In 2005 WHO produced a *Resource Book on Mental Health, Human Rights and Legislation* (WHO, 2005) which built on the MI Principles to provide guidelines for member states on the development of rights-based mental health legislation. In the era of global mental health human rights remain integral to the policies and guidelines of WHO and other actors and this has intensified with the advent of the UN Convention of the Rights of Persons with Disabilities (CRPD) (United Nations, 2006). The Convention has been ratified by nearly 200 countries worldwide, including Ghana, and describes wide-ranging and ambitious commitments to promoting and protecting the rights of persons with disabilities, including in this definition persons with mental illness, otherwise termed psychosocial disabilities. Where the MI Principles had focused on so-called 'negative rights', i.e. freedom from abuse, the Convention marked a new expansion of 'positive rights' to persons with mental illness by defining entitlements to political, economic, social and cultural rights.

However, the publication of the UN CRPD and subsequent campaigns surrounding its implementation highlighted a fundamental disjuncture between the language of human rights, self-determination and empowerment, and the practice of psychiatry in which involuntary treatment and detention remain a central aspect of treatment worldwide. Indeed the imbrication of psychiatry with the law has long been essential to its professional status as an arbiter on the management of perceived public safety and the control of mental illness. Although mental health law reform as promoted by the WHO (2005) is described as protecting human rights, for example by providing for courts of appeal for those confined, mental health laws worldwide, as in Ghana, are primarily used to legitimise coercive psychiatric treatment and appeals are rarely successful (Lund et al., 2012). The UN CRPD, on the other hand, has been promoted enthusiastically by mental health service-user organizations, who have interpreted it as outlawing all coercive treatment (Minkowitz, 2007). This has led to a criticism by psychiatrists who argue, like Osei, that involuntary treatment is essential to ensure 'the right to health' and prevent harm in cases where the person is judged to lack mental capacity (Freeman et al., 2015). The WHO has thus found itself in the uncomfortable position of promoting two contradictory positions under the banner of human rights (Wildeman, 2013).

Lunatics and confinement in British West Africa

Deinstitutionalization has been of less concern in the African continent, where historically most people with mental illness were not confined in asylums but remained in the care of the family or traditional healers (Collomb, 1975; Kilroy-Marac, 2019; Mahone, 2006; Swartz, 2010; Vaughan, 1991). Colonial administrators were markedly reluctant to establish asylums in the colonies, despite their popularity back home (Akyeampong, 2015),[3] and debates about the appropriate treatment of Africans with mental illness were inevitably refracted through colonialist ideologies. British colonial observers reported the common use of forms of restraint such as chains, shackles and logs for persons deemed mad in homes and traditional healing centres (Tooth, 1950; Cunyngham-Brown, 1937). However, even with such restraints care at home or from traditional healers was judged preferable to, and possibly more effective than, institutional confinement, and resonated with Lugard's 'dual mandate' to preserve traditional ways of life as well as to exert financial prudence (Heaton, 2013). In 1936 Dr Robert Cunyngham-Brown was tasked by the British government to inspect 'the care and treatment of lunatics' in their West African colonies. His first port of call was the then Gold Coast. Expecting to find most of the mentally ill confined in the asylum, he belatedly came to realise that most were in fact cared for either within the extended family or by 'native doctors'. He also examined fifty 'wandering lunatics'. In his final report Cunyngham-Brown eulogized the benefits of 'family care of the insane', which he viewed as 'a natural growth of age-long custom' and 'in entire harmony with the officially encouraged strengthening of native administrations' (Cunyngham-Brown, 1937: 24). He concluded that: 'The general attitude of the native peoples [...] to the vagrant lunatics [...] is one of kindly commiseration, tolerating much and giving alms as a matter of course [...] Elsewhere when visiting patients in their own homes, I found the same kindly bearing to the insane, and though many were chained or put in stocks, to my thinking often needlessly, it was evident that they were seldom neglected but instead were in receipt of kindly and assiduous though often ill-directed attention' (Cunyngham-Brown, 1937: 13).

Nonetheless, 'vagrant lunatics' in the growing urban centres were of concern to the colonial authorities. Fears of violence and public disorder were expressed by both colonial administrations and the public (Swartz, 2010). 'Alienation', the legal procedure for removing such persons from society, was inscribed into the British colonial legal apparatus through the implementation of 'lunacy ordinances' (Mahone, 2006; McCulloch, 1995; Quarshie, 2011–12).[4] Under 'indirect rule' village chiefs were responsible for reporting suspected cases of lunacy to the District Commissioners, who in turn requested examination by the Medical Officer. Once the case was deemed 'a proper subject for confinement' (Sadowsky, 1999), a 'certificate of alienation' was issued and the person could be removed. Initially those judged 'lunatic' were detained in prisons, although the need to provide spaces of confinement in tune with colonial humanitarian logic led to the establishment of a small number of dedicated asylums in cities such as Lagos, Freetown and Accra. However, their primary role concerned the management of public order, rather than therapy or rehabilitation (Quarshie, 2011–12; Sadowsky, 1999; Swartz, 2010).

Ghana (then the Gold Coast) was among the first of Britain's colonies to enact such procedures. The 1888 Lunatic Asylum Ordinance, modelled on the British legislation of the time, was drawn up 'to provide for the custody of lunatics' and permitted the detention, examination and 'certification' of persons suspected to be insane. Lunatics were imprisoned in a specially assigned wing of the Victoriaborg Castle in Accra before the construction of Accra asylum, now the psychiatric hospital, in 1906 (Quarshie, 2011–12). Most of those confined within the walls of colonial asylums had been removed from public spaces via the lunacy laws, and were often the most disturbed and destitute. There were very few medically qualified staff and little in the way of medical treatment (Akyeampong, 2015; Forster, 1962). Overcrowding, unsanitary conditions, as well as abuses of patients, including the use of mechanical restraint, were commonplace (de-Graft Aikins, 2015). Nonetheless, the possibility of forcibly removing dangerous or disturbed 'lunatics' to the asylum held some attraction both for families troubled by disruptive relatives and for authorities seeking to maintain public order and hygiene (de-Graft Aikins, 2015).

While the benefits of the family environment seemed to outweigh the indignity of chains in the family home, the common use of mechanical restraints and isolation cells in the few existing colonial asylums induced greater moral outrage among colonial observers. Such squalid surroundings and primitive methods within the heart of colonial institutions challenged the progressive view of colonialism's civilizing mission and threatened to discredit the colonial authorities (Heaton, 2013; Mahone, 2006; Sadowsky, 1999; Swartz, 2010). Cunyngham-Brown's inspection of Accra Lunatic Asylum in 1936 revealed severe overcrowding and several patients restrained in leg-irons and/or handcuffs or secluded 'on account of restlessness, violence and danger to others' (Cunyngham-Brown, 1937: 12). In contrast to his favourable impressions of the 'kindly' 'native peoples', Cunyngham-Brown was appalled at these conditions. He observed 'a noted reluctance on the part of both administrative and medical officers to send lunatics, if they are neither offenders nor dangerous, to an asylum which is known to be seriously over-crowded; preferring, indeed, as one medical officer told me, to return even such as would require mechanical restraint to the care of their families, as being more humane' (Cunyngham-Brown, 1937: 13).

Modernizing psychiatry in the independence era

By the mid-twentieth century asylums in the metropole had already fallen into disrepute and the disastrous impact of the two world wars on European economies put a break on ambitious infrastructural expansion in the colonies (Keller, 2005). The discovery of chlorpromazine's effects in calming psychosis in the early 1950s also coincided with the close of the colonial period and promised a new dawn for mental health care in which the perceived need for confinement could be substantially reduced. As countries moved to self-government in the post-war period the first African psychiatrists returned from training in Europe to head the psychiatric hospitals as modern institutions in keeping with the progressive vision of independent Africa. Most African psychiatrists from British colonies trained in the UK (Swartz, 2010), continuing a British influence on psychiatry which continues to the present. Where colonial psychiatry had emphasized a distinction between the 'native' and Western psyche, notably through Carothers' concept of the 'African mind', in which Africans were likened to children (Carothers, 1953), African psychiatrists argued not for difference but for equity (Heaton, 2013). The medicalization of madness in Africa formed a modernizing and professionalizing rhetoric which, as in Europe, was entwined with concerns about the most humane methods of restraint and treatment. Colonial law governing the care of lunatics remained in place, although responsibility for confinement moved from colonial medical officers to African psychiatrists. For African psychiatrists, their professionalization and efforts to appeal to the public also consisted in distinguishing themselves from traditional healers. This was not only in their exercise of scientific reasoning, but in their repudiation of inhumane methods of restraint.

Emmanuel Forster, a Gambian, was the first African psychiatrist to practise in Ghana. Trained in Britain, he was posted to the asylum, by then called Accra Mental Hospital, in 1951. Forster saw his role as bringing scientific reason and humane treatment and rescuing persons with mental illness from the 'charlatans' who punished patients considered to be 'agents of demons' (Forster, 1962: 25). His explicit contrast of 'scientific reason' with 'charlatan' healers is somewhat in opposition to those such as the Nigerian psychiatrist Thomas Lambo, who viewed traditional healers as sophisticated psychotherapists (Crosby, 1964).[5] Yet, despite his respect for their methods, even Lambo saw sedating psychotropics as preferable to healers' ropes and chains (Bass, 1997). As did Lambo, Forster saw the introduction of psychopharmaceuticals as central in transforming the hospital from a place of custody to a humane therapeutic environment. Importantly, restraint was now 'purely by chemical means', as opposed to the handcuffs and leg-irons previously in common use (Forster, 1962: 26). Patients were no longer solely brought in under the asylum ordinance, but increasing numbers were admitted at the request of their family. Notably, the practice of admitting 'vagrant psychotics' continued (de-Graft Aikins, 2015). As a consequence, the hospital was even more overcrowded after independence, with three times as many patients as beds. Nonetheless, Forster was optimistic about the future of psychiatry on the African continent and delineated a progressive vision in which psychiatry would expand to meet the growing demand arising from increasing awareness of its benefits (Forster, 1962).

In the years that followed two more psychiatric hospitals were constructed in Ghana; however, the flourishing of an African psychiatry as championed by Lambo and Forster was short lived. During the decades following independence African states, including Ghana, experienced political upheaval, with military coups and attacks on the socialist model adopted by many of Africa's new leaders, including the expansion of state-sponsored health care. The influence of the World Bank on health financing and the decline of the WHO shifted health policy from a humanitarian to an economic rationale (Pfeiffer and Chapman, 2010). Structural adjustment in the 1980s and 1990s took an enormous toll on publicly funded health systems in low-income countries (Akyeampong, Hill and Kleinman, 2015). Mental health, which was already extremely underfunded in comparison to other aspects of medical care, arguably suffered the most. Many doctors sent to train as psychiatrists overseas never returned. Throughout this period WHO policy continued to promote community-based mental health care and the integration of mental health within primary care, in keeping with the vision of Alma-Ata. However, for most African states this was an unattainable vision.

Global mental health in Ghana

Throughout the 1980s and 1990s, in the face of military coups, economic crisis, structural adjustment, famine and a mass exodus of health care professionals, the mental health system in Ghana, such as it was, struggled to survive. However, despite this unfavourable environment, during this period the seeds were sown for Ghana's later positioning at the vanguard of rights-based mental health reform in the region. One of the first acts of the military 'National Redemption Council' (NRC) in 1972 was to repeal the Lunacy Act and replace it with a Mental Health Decree. This had been drawn up under the previous civilian government with input from Dr Forster. The decree allowed for persons to be placed under 'care, observation and treatment' in a psychiatric hospital if assessed by a medical practitioner and 'there is good reason to believe the person in question to be suffering from mental illness, and that it is expedient for his welfare, or for the public safety'. The decree also mandated a Mental Health Review Tribunal under which persons could appeal against their detention, though this was never established. In addition, the NRC sponsored four Ghanaian doctors to train in psychiatry in the UK, one of whom, Joseph Asare, returned to Ghana and assumed the leadership of Accra Psychiatric Hospital in 1982. Joseph Asare was active in engaging with WHO projects, one of which was the WHO Nations for Mental Health (WHO, 2002), which attempted to implement the recommendations of the *World Mental Health* report (Desjarlais et al., 1995). As the name implies, this project was couched in ambitious terms which marked out its global scope, moving beyond individual nation-states to imagine a new 'nation' comprised of persons suffering from mental disorders and to 'create a world wide movement for mental health' (WHO, 2002). The programme brought together actors including the UN, the World Bank and NGOs to develop 'technical demonstration projects' and mobilise international attention to mental health. From the 1970s Ghana had begun posting psychiatric nurses to work in the community, and during the 1990s a number of psychiatric units were set up in regional hospitals. The Nations for Mental Health demonstration project in Ghana aimed to build on this to expand the provision of community-based mental health care. However, like many such projects, including the WHO Collaborative Study on Strategies for Extending Mental Health Care (Giel et al., 1983), which aimed to support the integration of mental health into primary care, the long-term effect was negligible, primarily due to a failure to mobilise ongoing funding and wider health system reform.

Since these beginnings Ghana's position as a node in the networks of global mental health has continued to expand. The return to democratic government in 1998 and economic growth have seen Ghana promoted as a model of democratic governance in the region, exemplary of the progressive narrative of 'Africa Rising'.[6] A number of international research projects have been conducted through collaborations with academics in the UK, South Africa and the US partnered by the WHO, the Disability Rights Fund and the UK Department for International Development (DFID) among others. International and local NGOs working in mental health have also been established, and the number continues to grow. In 2003 Dr Asare began discussions with the WHO to reform the mental health decree, and in 2006 a Mental Health Bill was drafted, informed by WHO guidance and with technical support from WHO personnel. The WHO hailed the Bill as a model for rights-based mental health legislation and supported advocacy campaigns for it to be passed into law. Dr Asare and his protégé Dr Osei, who took over as 'chief psychiatrist' in 2005, were astute in recruiting support from high-profile politicians, lawyers and international partners. Dr Osei in particular has been a tireless campaigner, appearing frequently in the media to advocate for mental health reform. However, negotiations to pass the Mental Health Bill were protracted, facing resistance from both the government and other actors in the health system. Pressure to pass the Bill intensified when HRW published a damning report exposing human rights abuses within the psychiatric hospital, Christian prayer camps and traditional shrines (Human Rights Watch, 2012). Shocking images of semi-naked people in chains and stories of people beaten, starved and neglected received widespread international media exposure. The Mental Health Act was finally passed in March 2012. The same year the UN CRPD was ratified by Ghana. Since then a number of NGOs have attracted international funding to campaign for the rights of persons with psychosocial disabilities and the implementation of the CRPD and the Mental Health Act. Increased numbers of community mental health workers are also being trained, with the aim to provide mental health services at every clinic in the country.

Enacting global mental health

Despite these efforts, the Mental Health Act has only partially been implemented. The passing of the Act occurred at a time when Ghana's economy began to enter a period of stagnation, in part a consequence of the global financial crisis. The price for securing International Monetary Fund loans has been a further reining in of public sector expenditure. The Mental Health Authority which was set up under the Act to provide administrative oversight for government mental health services has thus far been largely funded by DFID. At the time of writing the Mental Health Fund, mandated to fund mental health services, has not been established and the existing mental health budget is swallowed up by the three psychiatric hospitals. While there are more community mental health workers in post and they are more widely distributed through the country, there is no ring-fenced budget for their services, resulting in shortages of essential supplies, including psychopharmaceuticals. The visiting committees mandated by the Act to oversee the operations of 'unorthodox mental health care', such as traditional and Christian healers, have not been set up. Until 2018 the forms required for certificates of urgency had not been printed, meaning that Operation Clear the Streets was not as congruent with the law as Dr Osei claimed. Thus, in the years since its passing the Mental Health Act has not been as transformative as its proponents had hoped for. The routine chaining of persons with mental health problems continues in prayer camps, healers' shrines and family compounds, particularly in the north of the country (Guardian, 2020), leading to further criticism from rights-based organizations, including HRW and the UN Special Rapporteur on Torture, who visited the country in 2013 to report on conditions in the psychiatric hospitals, prayer camps and healers' shrines (Méndez, 2014). Local human rights actors, such as the Human Rights Advocacy Centre, have alleged that the state is in effect abdicating its responsibilities and 'institutionalising illegality' through its failure to intervene.

In stark contrast to the modern, air-conditioned offices of the Mental Health Authority, Accra Psychiatric Hospital remains in a state of advanced decay and is perhaps even less of a 'therapeutic community' than it was in the days of Emmanuel Forster. The crumbling walls topped with coils of rusting barbed wire stand in stark contrast to the glossy façade of the recently completed regional hospital only five minutes away. Near-constant funding crises mean that medical equipment, drugs, food and even detergents are in short supply. Unsurprisingly, 'Accra Mental', as the hospital is popularly known, is still largely perceived by the general public less as a place of therapy and rehabilitation than as one of confinement for the dangerously mad. Staff complain of families 'dumping' their relatives at the hospital and about the costs of supporting patients who are recovered but whose relatives cannot be traced. The mad vagrant still looms large in the public imaginary as a figure of social disintegration and moral transgression, whose presence on the streets threatens violence, dirt and disorder. Such a person, perhaps bewitched by a jealous rival or rendered mad through the breaking of taboos, commonly features in popular Ghanaian and Nigerian films, often portrayed in filthy, ragged clothing and with matted hair and staring eyes (Atilola and Olayiwola, 2013). Homeless persons on the streets are also often suspected to be using drugs, and thus to have intentionally removed themselves from society in order to pursue their particular vice. As a Ghanaian psychologist commented in 2016, the very condition of homelessness is, in the public imagination, synonymous with madness. Media reports often feature lurid tales of murder or assault perpetrated by persons who are mentally ill, including dismemberment and decapitation. Fears of persons with mental illness as aggressive, and the dangers of mad vagrants roaming in public spaces, tend to be reinforced rather than challenged by many working in mental health services, and even by attempts at publicly implementing the Mental Health Act, as was the case in Operation Clear the Streets. Despite its rights-based credentials, the Mental Health Act continues the principles of early lunacy ordinances and current mental health law in countries such as the UK in permitting the involuntary detention of 'Persons with mental disorder found in a public places' as Dr Osei describes. Such a person may be detained under a 'certificate of urgency' if the person is 'highly aggressive or showing out-of-control behaviour and appears to require immediate care, control and treatment' (Mental Health Act 2012, Act 846, Section 73). During one of the frequent nurses' strikes in 2016, the press reported public fears that violently aggressive patients would escape onto the streets. The nurses capitalized on the perceived dangerousness of their charges to argue for increased resources for the hospital. The nurses argued that it was a matter of 'public security' that the hospital be sufficiently funded. Indeed, one could see the underfunding of mental health services as contributing to the enduring use of coercion within the psychiatric hospital, where heavy sedation helps to allay fears of violence in settings where staff numbers are low and the built environment is unsanitary and unsafe (Jack et al., 2015).

Brokering human rights and mental health care

African psychiatrists such as Dr Osei thus find themselves caught between the vision of a humane, medically driven psychiatry in step with international human rights standards and the constraints of an underfunded public mental health system. Furthermore, to be relevant at home means answering to local demands for social control of persons with mental illness, while at the same time persuading the population of the validity (and humanity) of a medical perspective on mental disorders. This is rendered particularly challenging where psychiatric hospitals offer a less than appealing alternative in terms of effective treatment or humane options for confinement. The advent of global mental health and increased international funding and support has provided opportunities for some African psychiatrists and advocates to petition for reform. However, the tensions between the global vision of international agencies and local demands continue. Despite his comparison of Ghanaian and UK mental health law, Dr Osei has been keen to avoid accusations of neo-colonial dominance in the conceptualization of the human rights of persons with mental illness, an accusation that has been made in relation to lesbian and gay rights in Africa. By his own description, the Mental Health Act was a hybrid rather than a simple replication (Merry, 2006), which answered to international standards as well as local culture. The Act was, he said, 'synthesised, guided by the WHO, from the mental health laws of many countries with doses of Ghana's own culture. The law was, therefore, uniquely peculiar to Ghana's culture and not a replica of any country's law.'

In the absence of sustained government resources the performative spectacle (Miescher, Bloom and Manuh, 2014) of programmes such as Operation Clear the Streets makes the Mental Health Authority visible, both to international donors and global mental health actors and to local policy makers, philanthropists and the general public. In many ways, despite the international criticisms of Ghana's human rights record, Ghana's position in relation to globally comparative benchmarks of mental health care such as the WHO *Mental Health Atlas* (WHO, 2018) is rather better than that of some of its neighbours who have virtually no community mental health workers and whose legislation has not changed since the colonial era. The international attention Ghana has received in relation to human rights and mental health has enabled various government actors and NGOs to attract funding from DFID, the UN Fund for Victims of Torture and the Disability Rights Fund, among others. Much of this has been spent on activities to educate traditional and faith healers, or to purchase drug supplies and motorbikes for community mental health activities. However, the Mental Health Authority must also appeal to local benefactors, such as businesses and churches, several of whom have sponsored renovations of the psychiatric hospital infrastructure and whose donations maintain its day-to-day costs. Such internal support is vital, since, with global mental health policy committed to community-based services rather than inpatient care, psychiatric hospitals are less of a target for international donors, as Varma also describes in India (Cohen and Minas, 2017; Varma, 2016). Operation Clear the Streets, for example, received funds from the airport authority, who were keen to address the problem of vagrants hanging around the airport and its environs and sponsored the renovation of one of the hospital wards where they could be admitted.

By 2016 the operation had been renamed 'Restoring Dignity' to emphasise the rehabilitation of vagrants, although the technicalities remained unchanged. On the repainted 'vagrants' ward' a photograph album is kept as testimony to the transformation achieved through the programme. In the photographs, dishevelled homeless men are surrounded by hospital personnel in white coats while armed police stand by. One depicts a small mound of dried cannabis found in the possession of a vagrant. In another several nurses are pictured restraining a man while Dr Osei administers an injection into his upper arm. In another a man struggles as he is manhandled into a minibus emblazoned with 'Accra Psychiatric Hospital', his mouth stretched open, presumably loudly protesting his arrest. Side by side with these photos are shots taken after their rehabilitation, the person washed, their hair shaved, dressed in clean donated clothes. In the hospital a specialist team has been set up to trace patients' families and arrange for their return home, a process dubbed 'repatriation'. In the Mental Health Authority's annual report for 2017 'the removal, treatment and rehabilitation of eighty-three (83) vagrants' was explicitly framed as one of a number of 'human rights activities' which aimed to 'curb human rights abuses of persons with mental illness'. It claimed that 'A number of them who have recovered have been reintegrated into the community and united with their families' (Ghana Mental Health Authority, 2018).

However, as well as being internationally controversial, the repatriation programme has been less than entirely successful. Funds for the programme are sporadic, many families cannot be traced and some patients escape back onto the streets before they can be returned, as happened to one patient in 2016. Taken from the upmarket Accra Mall close to the airport, George had been brought to the hospital and treated. Tired of waiting for funds for a hospital bus to return him to his family, one day he disappeared, perhaps to his family or back onto the streets. Having stayed in the US, George was able to make an international comparison of his treatment and found Ghana wanting. For those who are returned home, the welcome they receive, sometimes after many years of absence, can only be guessed at. Accompanying social workers, a nurse and an NGO worker on a repatriation exercise in December 2018, I felt myself haunted by my own ethnography. In 2006, a year before global mental health was supercharged through the publication of the now infamous *Lancet* special issue (Lancet Global Mental Health Group, 2007), I had accompanied social workers from another psychiatric hospital on an identical mission, jolting along mud roads to remote villages to deposit long-lost vagrants in the homes of relatives. Then as now, each 'reintegration' took only a few minutes, involving the handing over of medication and instructions to the family to attend the nearest clinic for further supplies. While some families appeared to welcome the wanderer back with open arms, others appeared more ambivalent. Some families could not be found, either because the person could not identify their home or because the family had moved away. Many of those 'repatriated' clearly had grave social, physical or cognitive difficulties and would likely require ongoing support and care, both material and practical. These difficulties, combined with few employment opportunities, are likely to limit the chances of their returning to meaningful work and thus contributing to the household finances.

Conclusion

At first glance Operation Clear the Streets seems entirely incongruent with the high-minded aims of global mental health as articulated within the rights-based policies and programmes of international actors such as the WHO, UN and HRW. Yet calling forth the ghosts in the machine reveals the complex genealogies that have brought about this uneasy moment in the enactment of global mental health. These include the globalization of human rights through post-colonial networks of international agencies and local actors, disputed practices within the medico-legal governance of madness, colonial histories of confinement and post-colonial visions of modernizing mental health care, resource constraints and public sector retrenchment under neoliberal economic reforms, and popular moral concerns around vagrants, madness and violence. As Yarrow argues in respect of development projects in Ghana, seemingly universal forms such as 'human rights' are put to specific ends by particular actors within particular contexts. Within the situated enactment of global mental health, as for development, diverse forms of knowledge and ethics are assembled and reformulated (Yarrow, 2011: 124), leading to something that is not simply a local translation of a global ideal but a hybrid which attempts to simultaneously address global demands and local concerns. While Ghana's Mental Health Act is parsed as progress towards a modern mental health service, in the absence of sustained investment rather than intermittent donor-funded projects true transformation is constantly deferred. Rather, Operation Clear the Streets re-enacts historical practice in the guise of innovation.

Notes

1 'Health minister hails move to clear streets of mental patients, 13 May 2014, Ghanaweb, https://www.ghanaweb.com/GhanaHomePage/health/Health-Minister-hails-move-to-clear-streets-of-mental-patients-309169#.
2 This chapter draws primarily on anthropological research conducted by the author in Ghana for a total of five months in 2016, as well as documentary analysis of media and research reports and WHO archives. Other periods of research were conducted between 2006 and 2008 and in 2018. In 2016 observation and interviews were conducted with the assistance of Lionel Sakyi, University of Ghana, with staff, patients and family members from Accra Psychiatric Hospital. This included observation and interviews on the vagrants' ward. Ethical approval for the research was obtained from Ghana Health Service, Kwame Nkrumah University of Science and Technology and the University of Ghana Ethics Review Committees. Funding was provided by the Economic and Social Research Council (PTA-031-2005-00036), the European Research Council (340510) and the Wellcome Trust (203376/Z/16/Z).
3 The latter half of the nineteenth century inaugurated the 'asylum era' in Europe and the US, with the widespread expansion of custodial treatment and the introduction of 'lunacy ordinances' for the enforced detention of those deemed to be a danger to social order (Porter, 2006). However, there were significant differences in French and British colonial policy, to some extent reflecting colonial ideologies of assimilation on the part of the former and the 'White man's burden' on the part of the latter, as well the impact of domestic demands and world wars on colonial budgets (Keller, 2001). Although the British constructed a number of asylums in their African colonies from the end of the nineteenth century, including Accra Psychiatric Hospital, in French African territories, aside from Blida asylum in Algeria

constructed in the 1920s, dedicated psychiatric facilities were not constructed until the final decade of colonial rule (Collomb, 1975). Before then some of those with suspected mental illness were shipped to asylums in France. The Fann clinic in Senegal, established as a pioneering model of humane psychiatric care in the region, was inaugurated in 1956, just four years before the country gained independence (Kilroy-Marac, 2019).
4 Again, procedures in the French colonies took a rather different trajectory, although concerns regarding vagrancy and social order were common in both administrations. France did not apply asylum ordinances in its colonies and custody of the vagrant mentally ill was in prisons or general hospital annexes (Collomb, 1975). As in this case, in Senegal the entanglement of vagrancy with psychiatry extended into the post-colonial period (Collignon, 1984; Diagne, 2016).
5 Forster's rather dismissive attitude contrasts with others at the time, such as Patrick Twumasi, a sociologist, who compiled a seminal study of Ghana's medical systems. Like Lambo in Nigeria and the French psychiatrist Henri Collomb in Senegal (Collomb, 1973), he was a proponent of combining traditional healing with psychiatry (Twumasi, 1975).
6 The term 'Africa rising' has been widely deployed to reflect optimism about the growth in African economies, as in a 2011 article in *The Economist*, http://www.economist.com/node/21541015.

References

Akyeampong, E. (2015) 'A historical overview of psychiatry in Africa', in *The Culture of Mental Illness and Psychiatric Practice in Africa*, ed. Emmanuel Akyeampong, Allan G. Hill and Arthur Kleinman (pp. 24–49). Bloomington; Indianapolis: Indiana University Press.

Akyeampong, Emmanuel, Allan G. Hill and Arthur Kleinman (2015) 'Introduction: culture, mental illness, and psychiatric practice in Africa', in *The Culture of Mental Illness and Psychiatric Practice in Africa*, ed. Emmanuel Akyeampong, Allan G. Hill and Arthur Kleinman (pp. 1–23). Bloomington; Indianapolis: Indiana University Press.

Alem, Atalay and Catherine Manning (2016) 'Coercion in community mental health care: African perspectives', in *Coercion in Community Mental Health Care: International Perspectives*, ed. Andrew Molodynski, Jorun Rugkasa and Tom Burns (pp. 301–314). Oxford: Oxford University Press.

Atilola, O. and F. Olayiwola (2013) 'Frames of mental illness in the Yoruba genre of Nigerian movies: implications for orthodox mental health care', *Transcultural Psychiatry* 50 (3), 442–54. doi: 10.1177/1363461512443998.

Baasher, T., A. S. Elhakim, K. el Fawal, R. Giel, T. W. Harding and V. B. Wankiiri (1983) 'On vagrancy and psychosis', *Community Mental Health Journal* 19 (1), 27–41.
Bass, Thomas (1997) 'Traditional African psychotherapy: An interview with Thomas Adeoye Lambo', in *Magic, Witchcraft and Religion: An Anthropological Study of the Supernatural*, ed. A. C. Lehmann and J. E. Myers, pp. 165–170. Paolo Alto: Mayfield Publishing Company.
Brodwin, Paul and Livia Velpry (2014) 'The practice of constraint in psychiatry: emergent forms of care and control', *Culture, Medicine and Psychiatry* 38 (4), 524–526. doi: 10.1007/s11013-014-9402-y.
Carothers, John Colin (1953) *The African Mind in Health and Disease: A Study in Ethnopsychiatry*. Geneva: World Health Organization.
Cohen, A. and H. Minas (2017) 'Global mental health and psychiatric institutions in the 21st century', *Epidemiology and Psychiatric Sciences* 26 (1), 4–9. doi: 10.1017/S2045796016000652.
Collier, Stephen J. and Aihwa Ong (2005) 'Global assemblages, anthropological problems', in *Global Assemblages: Technology, Anthropology and Ethics as Anthropological Problems*, ed. Stephen J. Collier and Aihwa Ong (pp. 3–21). Malden, MA; Oxford; Victoria: Blackwell Publishing Ltd.
Collignon, René (1984) 'La lutte des pouvoirs publics contre les "encombrements humains" à Dakar', *Canadian Journal of African Studies/Revue canadienne des études africaines* 18 (3), 573–582. doi: 10.1080/00083968.1984.10804080.
Collins, P. Y., Vikram Patel, Sarah S. Joestl, Dana March, Thomas R. Insel, Abdallah S. Daar (2011) 'Grand challenges in global mental health', *Nature* 475 (7354), 27–30. doi: 10.1038/475027a.
Collomb, Henri (1973) 'Recontrer de deux systemes de soins. A propos de therapeutiques des maladies mentales en Afrique', *Social Science & Medicine* 7, 623–633.
Collomb, Henri (1975) 'Histoire de la psychiatrie en Afrique Noire Francophone', *African Journal of Psychiatry* 2, 87–115.
Cooper, Sara (2015) 'Prising open the "black box": an epistemological critique of discursive constructions of scaling up the provision of mental health care in Africa', *Health* 19 (5), 523–541. doi: 10.1177/1363459314556905.
Crosby, W. M. (1964) 'The village of Aro', *The Lancet* 2 (7358), 513–514.
Cunyngham-Brown, Robert (1937) *Report on Mission to the British Colonies of the West Coast of Africa on the Care and Treatment of Lunatics: The Gold Coast Colony*. London: Crown Agents.
de-Graft Aikins, Ama (2015) 'Mental illness and destitution in Ghana: a social-psychological perspective', in *The Culture of Mental Illness and Psychiatric Practice in Africa*, ed. Emmanuel Akyeampong, Allan G. Hill and Arthur

Kleinman (pp. 112–143). Bloomington; Indianapolis: Indiana University Press.

Desjarlais, Robert, Leon Eisenberg, Byron Good and Arthur Kleinman (1995) *World Mental Health: Problems and Priorities in Low-Income Countries*. New York; Oxford: Oxford University Press.

Diagne, Papa Mamadou (2016) 'Soigner les malades mentaux errants dans l'agglomération dakaroise. Socio-anthropologie de la santé mentale au Sénégal', *Anthropologie & Santé. Revue internationale francophone d'anthropologie de la santé* 13, http://journals.openedition.org/anthropologiesante/2171; DOI: https://doi.org/10.4000/anthropologiesante.2171.

Fakhoury, Walid and Stefan Priebe (2002) 'The process of deinstitutionalization: an international overview', *Current Opinion in Psychiatry* 15 (2), 187–192.

Forster, Emmanuel B. (1962) 'A historical survey of psychiatric practice in Ghana', *Ghana Medical Journal* 1 (1–2), 25–29.

Freeman, Melvyn C., Kavitha Kolappa, Jose M. de Almeida, Arthur Kleinman, Nino Makhashvili, Sifiso Phakathi, Bendetto Saraceno and Graham Thornicroft (2015) 'Reversing hard won victories in the name of human rights: a critique of the General Comment on Article 12 of the UN Convention on the Rights of Persons with Disabilities', *Lancet Psychiatry* 2 (9), 844–850. doi: 10.1016/S2215-0366(15)00218-7.

Ghana Mental Health Authority (2018) *2017 Annual Report*.

Giannakopoulos, George and Dimitris C. Anagnostopoulos (2016) 'Psychiatric reform in Greece: an overview', *Brithsh Journal of Psychiatry Bulletin* 40 (6), 326–328. doi: 10.1192/pb.bp.116.053652.

Giel, R., M. V. de Arango, A. Hafeiz Babikir, M. Bonifacio, C. E. Climent, T. W. Harding, H. H. Ibrahim, L. Ladrido-Ignacio, R. S. Murthy and N. N. Wig (1983) 'The burden of mental illness on the family. Results of observations in four developing countries. A report from the WHO Collaborative Study on Strategies for Extending Mental Health Care', *Acta Psychiatrica Scandinavica* 68 (3), 186–201.

Gostin, L. O (2008) '"Old" and "new" institutions for persons with mental illness: treatment, punishment or preventive confinement?' *Public Health* 122 (9), 906–913. doi: 10.1016/j.puhe.2007.11.003.

Guardian (2020) 'The scandal of Ghana's shackled sick', *Guardian*, 3 February.

Harding, T. (1973) 'Psychosis in a rural West African community', *Social Psychiatry* 8, 198–203.

Heaton, Matthew M. (2013) *Black Skin, White Coats: Nigerian Psychiatrists, Decolonization, and the Globalization of Psychiatry*. Athens: Ohio University Press.

Human Rights Watch (2012) 'Like a *death sentence*": abuses against persons with mental disabilities in Ghana. Human Rights Watch.

Jack, H., M. Canavan, E. Bradley and A. Ofori-Atta (2015) 'Aggression in mental health settings: a case study in Ghana', *Bulletin of the World Health Organization* 93 (8), 587–888. doi: 10.2471/BLT.14.145813.

Keller, R. (2001) 'Madness and colonialism: psychiatry in the British and French empires', 1800–1962, *Journal of Social History* 35 (2), 295–326.

Keller, R. C. (2005) 'Pinel in the Maghreb: liberation, confinement, and psychiatric reform in French North Africa', *Bulletin of the History of Medicine* 79 (3), 459–499. doi: 10.1353/bhm.2005.0112.

Kilroy-Marac, Katie (2019) *An Impossible Inheritance: Postcolonial Psychiatry and the Work of Memory in a West African Clinic*. Oakland, CA: University of California Press.

Kohn, Robert, S. Saxena, I. Levav and B. Saraceno (2004) 'The treatment gap in mental health care', *Bulletin of the World Health Organization* 82 (11), 858–866.

Lancet Global Mental Health Group (2007) 'Scale up services for mental disorders: a call for action', *The Lancet* 370 (9594), 1241–1252.

Lovell, A. M. and L. A. Rhodes (2014) 'Psychiatry with teeth: notes on coercion and control in France and the United States', *Culture, Medicine and Psychiatry* 38 (4), 618–622. doi: 10.1007/s11013-014-9420-9.

Lund, Crick, Tom Sutcliffe, Alan J. Flisher and Dan J. Stein (2012) 'Protecting the rights of the mentally ill in poorly resourced settings: Experiences from four African countries', in *Mental Health and Human Rights, Vision, Praxis and Courage*, ed. Michael Dudley, Derrick silove and Fran Gale (pp. 527–537). Oxford: Oxford University Press.

Mahone, Sloan (2006) 'Psychiatry in the East African colonies: a background to confinement', *International Review of Psychiatry* 18 (4), 327–332. doi: 10.1080/09540260600859621.

McCulloch, Jock (1995) *Colonial Psychiatry and 'The African Mind'*. Cambridge: Cambridge University Press.

Méndez, Juan E. (2014) *Report of the Special Rapporteur on torture and other cruel, inhuman or degrading treatment or punishment. Addendum, Mission to Ghana*. United Nations General Assembly Human Rights Council Twenty-fifth Session.

Merry, Sally Engle (2006) 'Transnational human rights and local activism: mapping the middle', *American Anthropologist* 108 (1), 38–51.

Miescher, Stephan, Peter J. Bloom and Takyiwaa Manuh (2014) 'Introduction', in *Modernization as Spectacle in Africa*, ed. Peter J. Bloom, Stephan Miescher, Takyiwaa Manuh and Percy C. Hintzen (pp. 1–16). Bloomington: Indiana University Press.

Minkowitz, T. (2007) 'The United Nations Convention on the Rights of Persons with Disabilities and the right to be free from noncensensual psychiatric interventions', *Syracuse Journal of International Law and Commerce* 34 (2), 405–428.

Molodynski, Andrew, Jorun Rugkasa and Tom Burns (eds) (2016) *Coercion in Community Mental Health Care: International Perspectives*. Oxford: Oxford University Press.

Murthy, S. R. (2001) 'Lessons from the Erwadi tragedy for mental health care in India', *Indian Journal of Psychiatry* 43 (4), 362–366.

Patel, V., B. Saraceno and A. Kleinman (2006) 'Beyond evidence: the moral case for international mental health', *American Journal of Psychiatry* 163 (8), 1312–1315. doi: 10.1176/ajp.2006.163.8.1312.

Pfeiffer, James and Rachel Chapman (2010) 'Anthropological perspectives on structural adjustment and public health', *Annual Review of Anthropology* 39 (1), 149–165. doi: 10.1146/annurev.anthro.012809.105101.

Porter, Roy (2006) *Madmen: A Social History of Madhouses, Mad-Doctors and Lunatics*. Stroud: Tempus Publishing Limited. Original edition, 1987.

Quarshie, Nana (2011–12) 'Confinement in the luncatic asylums of the Gold Coast from 1887–1906', *Psychopathologie Africaine* XXXVI (2), 1–35.

Sadowsky, Jonathan (1999) *Imperial Bedlam: Institutions of Colonial Madness in Southwest Nigeria*. Berkeley: University of California Press.

Saya, A., C. Brugnoli, G. Piazzi, D. Liberato, G. Di Ciaccia, C. Niolu and A. Siracusano (2019) 'Criteria, procedures, and future prospects of involuntary treatment in psychiatry around the world: a narrative review', *Fronters in Psychiatry* 10 (271). doi: 10.3389/fpsyt.2019.00271.

Scheper-Hughes, N. and A. M. Lovell (1986) 'Breaking the circuit of social control: lessons in public psychiatry from Italy and Franco Basaglia', *Social Science & Medicine* 23 (2), 159–178.

Street, Alice (2018) 'Ghostly ethics', *Medical Anthropology* 37 (8), 703–707. doi: 10.1080/01459740.2018.1521400.

Swartz, S. (2010) 'The regulation of British colonial lunatic asylums and the origins of colonial psychiatry, 1860–1864', *History of Psychology* 13 (2), 160–177.

Testa, Megan and Sara G. West (2010) 'Civil commitment in the United States', *Psychiatry* 7 (10), 30–40.

Thornicroft, Graham and Paul Bebbington (1989) 'Deinstitutionalisation – from hospital closure to service development', *British Journal of Psychiatry* 155 (6), 739–753. doi: 10.1192/bjp.155.6.739.

Thornicroft, Graham and Michele Tansella (2004) 'Components of a modern mental health service: a pragmatic balance of community and hospital care:

overview of systematic evidence', *British Journal of Psychiatry* 185, 283–290. doi: 10.1192/bjp.185.4.283.

Tooth, Geoffrey (1950) *Studies in Mental Illness in the Gold Coast*, Colonial Research Publications no. 6. London: H.M.S.O.

Tsing, Anna Lowenhaupt (2005) *Friction: An Ethnography of Global Connection*. Princeton, NJ; Woodstock: Princeton University Press.

Twumasi, Patrick A. (1975) *Medical Systems in Ghana: A Study in Medical Sociology*. Accra: Ghana Publishing Corporation.

United Nations (1991) *Principles for the Protection of Persons with Mental Illness and the Improvement of Mental Health Care*. Office of the High Commissioner for Human Rights, Resolution 46/119.

United Nations (2006) *Convention on the Rights of Persons with Disabilities and Optional Protocol*. New York: United Nations.

Varley, Emma and Saiba Varma (2018) 'Spectral ties: hospital hauntings across the line of control', *Medical Anthropology* 37 (8), 630–644. doi: 10.1080/01459740.2018.1490280.

Varma, Saiba (2016) 'Disappearing the asylum: modernizing psychiatry and generating manpower in India', *Transcultural Psychiatry* 53 (6), 783–803. doi: 10.1177/1363461516663437.

Vaughan, Megan (1991) *Curing Their Ills: Colonial Power and African Illness*. Oxford: Polity Press.

WHO (2001) *The World Health Report 2001: Mental Health: New Understanding, New Hope*. Geneva: World Health Organization.

WHO (2002) *Nations for Mental Health: Final Report*. Geneva: World Health Organization, Mental Health Policy and Service Development, Department of Mental Health and Substance Dependence.

WHO (2005) *WHO Resource Book on Mental Health, Human Rights and Legislation*. Geneva: World Health Organization.

WHO (2007) Ghana country summary, in *Mental Health Improvement for Nations Development (MIND)*. Geneva: Department of Mental Health and Substance Abuse.

WHO (2018) *Mental Health Atlas 2017*. Geneva: World Health Organization.

Wildeman, S. (2013) 'Protecting rights and building capacities: challenges to global mental health policy in light of the Convention on the Rights of Persons with Disabilities', *Journal of Law, Medicine & Ethics* 41 (1), 48–73. doi: 10.1111/jlme.12005.

Yarrow, Thomas (2011) *Development Beyond Politics: Aid, Activism and NGOs in Ghana*. Basingstoke: Palgrave Macmillan.

Zigon, Jarrett (2010) 'Moral and ethical assemblages: A response to Fassin and Stoczkowski', *Anthropological Theory* 10 (1–2), 3–15.

6

You've got the point? Acupuncture and the techno-politics of bodyscape

Wen-Hua Kuo

Learn the rules like a pro, so you can break them like an artist. (Attributed to Pablo Picasso)

Introduction: global acupuncture and bodies on treatment

Acupuncture is an essential part of East Asian medicine. A peculiar way of diagnosing and treating people via meridians inside their bodies punctuated by regulatory points, it is a simple yet sophisticated art of healing that has been used for thousands of years. To appreciate acupuncture, beginning acupuncturists have to start with the rules, meaning they need to memorize the names and locations of acupuncture points and the meridians to which they belong before practising acupuncture on the human body. As in any bodily therapeutics, skills involving placing needles and manipulating them emerge as a passage toward *de qi* (bring about the desired sensation), the transcendental harmony between the healer and the healed.

After circulating in East Asia for more than 1,000 years, acupuncture was introduced into Europe in the late seventeenth century as an oriental way of healing, and some personal efforts to promote this art were made in the early twentieth century (Candelise, 2008; Lu and Needham, 2002). Even so, it was US President Richard Nixon's historic visit to China in 1971 that opened up not only the communist People's Republic of China (PRC) but also – via acupuncture – the treasure box of traditional Chinese medicine (TCM).[1] The interest in acupuncture also led to an influx of TCM physicians into the US during the turmoil of the Chinese Cultural Revolution.

Acupuncture also influenced public health at the global level. Following its recognition of traditional medicine in 1979 by listing 208 medicinal herbs as essential to a country's public health, the WHO went on to proclaim that acupuncture should be taken seriously as a treatment of significant value. In addition to some instances of medical aid that incorporate TCM or other East Asian medicines, a twenty-first-century example of using acupuncturists to facilitate global health can be best demonstrated by the non-profit organization Barefoot Acupuncturists, which was founded by Belgian acupuncturist Walter Fischer in 2009. Inspired by the PRC's barefoot doctor movement in the 1960s and 1970s, this organization aims to provide efficient and affordable care with acupuncture in Mumbai and has treated more than 4,500 patients in India.[2]

Meanwhile, acupuncture attracts biomedical scrutiny through its global spread. Such efforts date back to early encounters between East and West, as seen in an introductory paper in *The Lancet* in 1823 (Lock, Last and Dunea, 2001: 9). However, serious appraisal of its use in pain control did not appear until the late 1940s. George Soulie de Morant (1879–1955), a long devotee of acupuncture in France, published *L'Acuponcture Chinoise* (1951), which was widely used by his European followers, including: Eric H. Wilhelm Stiefvater, the author of *Akupunktural und Neuraltherapie* (1956); Paul Nogier, the reviver of auriculotherapy; and Reinhold Voll, the inventor of Elektroakupunkturnach Voll. Compared to other traditional clinical practices in East Asia, such as herbal formulas and massage, acupuncture is uniquely Asian, yet rational to the rest of the world.

Acupuncture's popularity as described above can be explained by what historian of Chinese science Joseph Needham called 'grand titration' (1969). According to Needham, science and technology, no matter where they are orientated, belong to human civilization. A historian's job, like a chemist practising titration, is to consider scientific and technological innovations, piece by piece, as part of the flow of cultural activities that form the advancement of human culture. Although early uses of acupuncture can be found in ancient Egypt and India, it was East Asia that granted acupuncture theoretical frames and disseminated it globally.

Departing from this transcultural yet linear narrative that presumes a unified ladder of biomedical science and its alternatives, this chapter is interested in acupuncture's travels and the discrepancies emerging on its journey through cultures.[3] Pioneering authors addressing traditional medicines in the modern world include Elisabeth Hsu (1999) and Volker Scheid (2002), who discussed TCM in contemporary China. Recent literature has followed the dissemination of TCM throughout the world (such as Scheid and MacPherson, 2012; Zhan, 2009), noting the cultural and social aspects of its spread in places where it has been considered an alternative to biomedicine. In the end, the medicine which we call 'Chinese', as historian of medicine Charlotte Furth puts it, 'emerges as a pluralistic system with global reach involving complex accommodations with local medical cultures and institutions both at home and abroad' (Furth, 2011: 5).

On the other hand, the bodies that call for treatment are diverse. In addition to explorations on the different conceptualizations of the body in culture and in history (to name a few, Duden, 1991; Kuriyama, 1999; Laqueur, 1992; Lock, 1993, 2002), the differentiation of the body as a corporeal existence of culture does not cease in the wake of biomedicine's prevalence.[4] Margaret Lock and Vinh-Kim Nguyen (2010), for example, called attention to local biologies, which opens bodily and conceptual possibilities against the universality of the body brought by biomedicine. They claim: 'Understanding the body as contextually situated means that we attribute variations in biology to regularities produced by temporal process rather than to statistical laws' (Lock and Nguyen, 2010: 108). Unlike the biomedical understanding of the body that treats bodily differences as variations according to the presumption that all bodies are fundamentally similar, Lock and Nguyen remind us of the process of making such regularities, a process that makes such differences 'manifest as a predictable, a-temporal, "normal" distribution' (Lock and Nguyen, 2010: 108).

Guided by the notion of making regularities on the body, as Margaret Lock would call it in the making of biomedicine, this chapter starts its investigation with the names and locations of acupuncture points and the essential rules of acupuncture. In spite of their apparent simplicity and straightforwardness, the global journey of these points is not a process of translation from one language to another. For example, in *L'Acuponcture Chinoise* Morant listed the acupuncture points of the

Acupuncture and the techno-politics of bodyscape 133

head section of the stomach meridian, whose order is different from that used in the US and Asia. Paul Nogier, who proclaimed a somatic correlation between different anatomical areas of the body and specific points on the ear, differed from Chinese doctors, who learned of Nogier's diagram in the 1950s and developed their own diagram according to TCM theory (Rubach 2001 [1995]).

Some mistranslations read harmless. As TCM expert Deshen Wang pointed out (1987), early Westerners used the Wades-Giles Romanization system and ignored the fact that some characters have several readings (such as the character '俞', which should be read as 'shu' instead of 'yu' when used in acupuncture points). Some people misrecognized Chinese characters and, as a result, their romanization was incorrect.[5] Nonetheless, in some cases the inconsistent naming or ordering of acupuncture points, such as the order of the stomach meridian points mentioned above, can be controversial according to the meridian theory.[6] For practitioners, the method of naming these points implies a particular understanding of their function and use in healing.

Techno-politics in making regularities for global acupuncture

The price that traditional medicine pays in order to be globally accessible is more than inevitable plurality through dissemination. As with any translation, confusions and contradictions emerge, depending on the context in which traditional medicines are introduced and developed. In his study of TCM in Republican China, Sean Hsiang-lin Lei (2014) nicely used the period phrase 'neither donkey nor horse' to describe the political/epistemic limbo of TCM when attempting to incorporate biomedicine. In the same vein, Eunjeong Ma and Michael Lynch (2014) argued that the boundary between biomedicine and Korean medicine is not hard and fast and keeps changing, with practitioners of the latter now attempting to incorporate the imaging technology of computed tomography into their practice. The translatability of technologies, as they have claimed, changes according to the context of disputes over the scope and nature of Korean medicine.

What complicate the East/West dichotomy in healing are the boundaries among medical traditions in East Asia, where herbal formulas, therapeutic methods and healing philosophies have been exchanged for thousands of years. Compared to its division from biomedicine,

TCM shares terms and ideologies, via Chinese characters, with other examples of 'oriental medicine', such as Japan's *kampo* and Korea's *dongyi*. Even so, the resemblance of these components does not make these medicines more similar. Shaped during the period when these countries were seeking modernization, these medical traditions are often claimed to be highly original and distinct from other traditions in this region.

The landscape described above challenged Needham's titration thesis, where the task ends with the insertion of the non-biomedical into the developmental narrative of an ecumenical medicine (Kuo, 2019). In fact, the puzzle for health policy makers and for those who believe in the scientific merit of acupuncture is how to make it a part of the existing therapeutic repertory. Before doing so, one problem they have to deal with is fundamental: how to properly identify acupuncture points, and how to make sure that, when worked by different people, one point refers to the same location on the body.

Therefore, focusing on intellectual/diplomatic actions in the regularity setting, this chapter is a critical assessment of two attempts to standardize acupuncture undertaken by the WHO, the first relating to nomenclature between 1983 and 1989 and the second relating to acupuncture point location between 2003 and 2008. For those who struggle with acupuncture's terminologies, standardization has the merit of not only summarizing an enormous amount of precise and cumulative experience but also serving as the basis for future studies that will make acupuncture scientific. The standard created thus serves both as a master version of acupuncture on which all practices are based while considering its variations in different cultures, and as a corporeal bridge for this healing art to biomedicine.

Even with these good intentions, the making of such a standard did not go smoothly. The experts involved made clear their reservations regarding the standard they had created. For the public, this endeavour is most remembered for the quarrel between Korea and the PRC as to whose standard should be adopted as the global standard.[7] Complicating the otherwise generic political account that refers to the result as a consequence of geopolitics among East Asian states, this chapter highlights its technological aspect, arguing that scientific standard making is a techno-political endeavour in which science is always debated and shaped as a part of social interactions. Instead of portraying how experts lost their disinterestedness to allow nationalism to 'contaminate' the spirit of acupuncture, this chapter aims to demonstrate how these experts, with their diverse perceptions of the body as it relates to the umbrella of acupuncture, attempted to find bodily and lexical common ground.

Two approaches, one literary and the other philosophical, are useful for understanding this process. The first concerns the nature of debate over translations. Analysing the making of standard TCM terminologies, Sonya E. Pritzker (2014) suggested that such a process be considered 'in a broader field of "translation" as a dynamic human process', in which language matters in bringing up relationships between people involved, imagined relationships between China and the West and 'relationships between a desired other and experiential self' (Pritzker, (2014: 37–38). Projecting this situation as what Mikhail Bakhtin called 'heteroglossia', Pritzker also referred to standard making as 'a translingual practice', a concept created by literary theorist Lydia Liu (1995). Liu, by rejecting the separation of translation from society, claimed that '[T]he study of translingual practice examines the process by which new words, meanings, discourses, and modes of representation arise, circulate, and acquire legitimacy within the host language due to, or in spite of, the latter's contact/collision with the guest language' (Liu, 1995: 26). In accordance with the viewpoints presented in these studies, this chapter follows the experts and their meetings, or 'occasions', in using Liu's terms to capture the acupuncture point standards written in the universal academic language of English. More importantly, unlike Pritzker's case study, which looks only at the terms being discussed, this chapter pays equal attention to the forms, styles and ways in which the standards are composed, which also matter in translingual practice.

Furthering the idea of treating standard acupuncture points as a text, the second approach highlights their bodily aspect, suggesting the standards to be a bodyscape that should be read as a map. Starting with Bruno Latour's notion of 'immutable mobile' (Latour, 1986), according to which information is 'fixed', such as on maps, to be passed among agents, substantial literature exists in Science, Technology and Society (STS) to study maps as visual artefacts that represent both space and social relations (Harley, 1988; Knorr-Cetina and Amann, 1990) and as objects that invoke the users' attention in their everyday practices (Vertesi, 2008). In particular, concerning the problem of representation in science, Sergio Sismondo and Nicholas Chrisman's analysis on realism (2001) provides us with necessary guidance. Using a map as both a metaphor and a means of interpretation, they established a metaphysical frame for approaching reality based on deflationary philosophy, arguing that scientific representations are maps embedded in a particular kind of practice and for a particular use. The standard for acupuncture points can be understood in this way. By working on the multilingual versions of acupuncture, this chapter approaches standardization as a 'reversed engineering' of maps, during which the standard created is neither a social construction nor a real reflection of reality. It is, after all, a scientific representation – a textual/visual solution shaped by practice and allowing different readings.

Investigating the two WHO projects in making acupuncture universal and regular, this chapter addresses the understanding of acupuncture points before the 1980s and the institutional efforts made in the area of standardization. It then turns to the project of nomenclature, investigating how names became the target for standardization, with a glossary of acupuncture points being composed and the names of meridians determined.

The second part of this chapter deals with the standardization of acupuncture point locations in the first decade of the twenty-first century. The political landscape of East Asia may have hugely changed between the two projects; however the techno-politics within the expert meetings did not. Rather than debating these versions of acupuncture and choosing one where agreement existed, the standard produced was the result of a hybrid of languages, some classical, some scientific and some created for the purpose of standardization. In addition, instructions, instead of illustrations, became central to this standard. This is very different from the titration analogy, in which the task of standardization might simply involve turning the clock of evolution back, finding the 'origin' and resuming the process of modernization from there. Instead, what emerged from the long negotiations among these experts is a representational foundation onto which transcultural versions could be attached retrospectively as variations.

Rectifying names and creating a glossary: the 1980s nomenclature

By the early 1980s various theories had been developed to find a bodily foundation for meridians and acupuncture points. As the renowned acupuncture researcher Weibo Zhang summarizes (2012), from the perspective of energy flow these theories emphasize reactions rather than conventional routes of qualifying meridians. They identify acupuncture points from surrounding tissues through their distinct thermal, electrical and magnetic behaviours.

Among these theories, the theory of 'good conductors' (*ryodoraku*) is pioneering.[8] Ryodoraku was developed by Yoshio Nakatani at Kyoto University in 1951. He found a series of low electrical resistance points (*ryodoten*, electro-permeable points) running longitudinally up and down the body. By measuring these points and linking them together as ryodoraku lines, Nakatani claims that these lines closely match acupuncture meridians.[9] Without further proof to show the similarity between the two, in the decades that followed ryodoraku served as a theoretical basis for scientific research on acupuncture and diagnostic instruments for clinical use.

Nomenclature is another aspect of the inconsistency in acupuncture. Not only do Japan and Korea use different Chinese characters for some acupuncture points, but Europeans developed their own means of romanization. They developed a coding system to promote acupuncture beyond the Sinophone circle. For example, Quchi (LI 11), the 11th regulatory point in the Large Intestine meridian, can be codified as 'DCh$_{11}$' (PRC); 'II 11' (Japan); 'Li$_{11}$' (UK); 'GI 11' (France); 'Di 11' (Germany); or 'LI 11' (US). This problem was identified in the 1960s when the first world conference on acupuncture and moxibustion was held. However, until their sixth meeting in Paris in 1979 no further actions were taken.[10]

Meanwhile, the PRC established their own method of naming acupuncture points. As a national policy, a Chinese style of romanization – Hanyu Pinyin – was imposed in 1958 and began to be used by Western acupuncture students after 1972. In 1977 the UN decided that Hanyu Pinyin was the standard for the romanization of place names in China. Following that decision, the PRC government extended this policy to Chinese personal names in 1978.

As the PRC gradually appeared in international acupuncture landscapes,[11] the need to establish a universal standard was clear.[12] Urged by Japan, an independent committee on the standardization of meridians and points was formed in 1974. The members included Australia and the Asian states of Korea and the Philippines. Japan also conducted a survey of acupuncture classics in 1978. Finally, with the introduction of the WHO, four expert meetings between Japan and the PRC were held from 1981 to 1982. These meetings established the structure of the decision-making process for WHO projects: not all UN member states have an equal voice. With acupuncture recognized as an 'Asian' topic, nine states from the WHO's West Pacific Region – Japan, the PRC, Korea, Hong Kong, Australia, the Philippines, New Zealand, Singapore and Vietnam – were invited as stakeholders to discuss the draft before sending it to headquarters for approval.

On the surface, limiting the states involved to those in the 'Chinese character cultural sphere' seemed to simplify the task. These experts needed to clarify the locations of acupuncture points as described in *The Emperor's Inner Canon* (Huangdi Neijing), the authoritative source of acupuncture, and to give them proper names. However, in reality this arrangement encountered difficulties by sharpening the contrasts among Asian states in interpreting the classics with modern terms.

Japan, for example, proposed the idea of basic lines to locate acupuncture points. For regions that lack anatomical landmarks for identifying points, such as chest and abdomen, Akio Debata suggested using a grid-like accessory as a reference. Although this idea had appeared as early as the second Sino-Japanese expert meeting and had been debated throughout the standardization process, Chinese experts consistently had reservations. They claimed that they were not the original references (i.e. meridians) and were redundant. As the standardization of acupuncture point locations was postponed, this idea was finally turned down as the standard neared completion.

The PRC, on the other hand, hoped to use simplified Chinese characters and a Chinese phonetic alphabet (Hanyu Pinyin) for the names of acupuncture points. Like a Chinese–English dictionary, each point had a corresponding explanation as to its meaning. According to the proposal, this arrangement was intended to preserve the origin of acupuncture while remaining user friendly for those who do not read Chinese characters. However, for other Asian states it would create a situation where the PRC had the only 'gateway' for acupuncture users via its characters and the romanization system. In the end, an alphanumeric code replaced Hanyu Pinyin as the leading name for each acupuncture point, and no authorized explanations were provided to interpret them.

With the above concerns in mind, we know why the WHO project of the 1980s proposed so much but delivered so little in terms of a common standard. Kiichiro Tsutani, the coordinator of the WHO project at the time, recalled that it was a cultural challenge for East Asia, as they lacked experience in harmonizing standards.[13] Aside from determining the scope of the work process for discussion, the names of the meridians and acupuncture points were the only elements that everyone could agree on.

Even the rectification of these names was problematic. Concerning the acupuncture points, the PRC initially proposed simplified Chinese characters but did not insist on having them included in the standard. However, opposition from Japan, Korea and Vietnam meant that traditional Chinese characters in their 'original form' were chosen. As a result, simplified Chinese was selected as just one of the East Asian versions among Japanese *kanji* and Korean *hanja*. At the PRC's insistence, Hanyu Pinyin became the standard romanization for acupuncture points. Even so, occurring without any explanation, these names are very arbitrary and it is difficult to trace their linguistic origin.

Interestingly, in the case of meridian names, Japan and Korea suggested using English translations instead of Pinyin romanization. Claiming to respect those who had been using English when naming meridians (for example, GB is the abbreviation for 'Gall Bladder', referring to the gall bladder meridian), these experts wanted to follow this nomenclature and add eight extra meridians. In this case they would take the risk of misinterpretation and go against the PRC's 'dictionary' approach of standard making, which called the Triple Energizer meridian and the Thoroughfare Vessel 'Sanjiao' and 'chongmai', respectively. The controversy remained till the final meeting in Geneva, where the TCM authority Paul Unschuld was invited to settle the debate; he did so by validating the translations.

As a result, this 1980s WHO project produced a glossary rather than a standard. People might think it is a rational step toward standardization and that the rectification of names is a basic step. However, as shown in this section, that is not quite the case. Given its techno-political context, it was an evitable outcome of a translingual practice. In reality, the experts did not clarify the meanings of these points before giving them formal names. Neither did they validate the meridians before allowing them be referenced for acupuncture point locations. The first step of a translingual practice, as pointed out by Lydia Liu in her study on the introduction of Western concepts into Chinese, is the creation of a glossary. This list of terminology is not a translation of the host language, Liu insists, but altogether new terms. They are shorthand for concepts that are not yet fully understood in guest languages.

The standard acupuncture nomenclature provides such a glossary. The 'host language', being traditional Chinese, has disappeared from participating states.[14] As a reference, it is used to lay out its various versions in guest languages. The glossary does not guarantee that each corresponding term has equal meaning; rather, it only puts them together. Using the metaphor of a map, the function of this glossary becomes clear. Rejecting controversial interpretations, this glossary reads like a bus map. It has names of routes and stops on them. To use it, readers have to have knowledge of where these stops are. Yet the tricky thing remains: for the 'invisible city' of acupuncture, which body does this map refer to?

Making the body readable: the 2000s standard acupuncture point locations

It would be nearly two decades after the development of this standardized nomenclature before the idea of standardizing acupuncture point location was introduced in 2002 by Ken Chen, who at the time was the WHO Western Pacific Region Office (WPRO) officer on traditional medicine. Although some guidelines were created in the 1990s, including those on Basic Training and Safety in Acupuncture and those on Clinical Research on Acupuncture, they failed to address the most fundamental question in acupuncture: where exactly are the locations discussed – these places where the practitioners' needles are inserted?

Seung-hoon Choi, the successor of Ken Chen and the coordinator of this project, felt confident when he received this task. He recalled in an interview that some threads of discussion had touched upon the first standardization,[15] for example adopting the East Asian way of measuring acupuncture points[16] and respecting the way in which classic texts approach this issue. In addition, the WHO had learned how to set up procedures, making sure that the PRC, Japan and Korea could reach consensus before sending the standard to other WHO member states for approval. Ambitious and shrewd, Choi recognized the value of a global standard and believed that he could complete it with just three meetings.

After a preview meeting of experts in Manila to summarize the outstanding problems in the 1980s standardization and the tasks to be achieved, the first expert meeting was held in March 2004 in Beijing, where a principle for standardization, the so-called 'Beijing consensus', was formed.[17] According to this principle, with the slogan 'respect history and reality', the location of acupuncture points has to be faithful to the descriptions in the classics and can be expressed not purely by terms in traditional medical texts but in anatomical terms.

Superficially this appeared to be another task of translating acupuncture classics into a modern description. However, in reality it proved to be much more complicated than Choi had expected. Shortly after they met, the experts found that the classics could be problematic and confusing. For example, they recognized that *The Emperor's Inner Canon* did not identify all acupuncture points, but no consensus had yet been reached on what additional classics should be included as reference works. The PRC recommended a reconstructed version of a first-century classic, *The Yellow Emperor's Mingtang Classic* (Huangdi Mingtang Jing), but this was disqualified as not an original text. The Korean and Japanese experts suggested instead *The Great Compendium of Acupuncture and Moxibustion* (Zhen Jiu Jiayi Jing), the earliest existing classic on acupuncture in the sixth century. In the end, both were selected as reference works.

The interpretation of these classics also created problems. As an inseparable component of the healing tradition, these books have been annotated and intensively debated for centuries. Some acupuncture points have several names and some names refer to multiple locations. More importantly, no interpretations of the classic texts are universally accepted; rather, they are diverse and have been blended into the medical culture where they are generated, circulated and mixed with other therapeutics. Therefore, it is not surprising that, out of the 361 meridian acupuncture points, there were discrepancies of approach in the case of 92 points used in the PRC, Korea and Japan. Anatomy could not settle such huge discrepancies. Instead, it was supposed to provide descriptions, functioning like footnotes to the main text, after the ultimate interpretations had been determined.

For these problems, STS studies have shed some light, if we consider standards a literary technology of science (Shapin and Schaffer, 1985). Citing again Lydia Liu's notion of translingual practice (1995), in which she argues that novelistic realism in China should not be naively taken as reflecting social life in the 1930s, these works should be assessed in the first instance according to their narrative style and figuration. In particular, Liu suggests a reading of these works that takes seriously the traces of 'productive distortion', in which eloquent witness is disguised by seemingly parodic imitation (Liu, 1995: 103). Although anatomical terms have eventually been woven into acupuncture classics to describe the locations of acupuncture points, the standard should not be read as a cheap copy of biomedicine as imposed onto acupuncture. In the light of the translingual practice of bodyscape, I argue that the standards offer eloquent witness of the techno-politics surrounding their creation.

Like all literary work, the process of creating standards is painful. After the experts agreed on the languages that would be used in the standards (anatomical landmarks,[18] the traditional bodily approach to points[19] and relative measurement units in acupuncture classics), Choi informally divided them into groups, one on the interpretation of classics and the other on anatomical descriptions. The divergence at stake was not the distinction between 'East/West' or between 'traditional/modern'. Instead, it was a result of the differences within the three Asian states where some sort of national standards had existed. Whereas Korea had established its standards using anatomical terms, Japan and the PRC relied more on a traditional bodily approach. Moreover, compared to Japan and Korea, where national standards had been a part of their profession, the PRC's national standard was still in the process of consolidation. All these differences contributed to frictions among these experts and affected how the standard was composed.

Taking each acupuncture point as independent of the other points, the task in the following expert meetings turned out to be that of dissolving the discrepancies among the three states, point by point. Nigel Wiseman, a veteran TCM interpreter, was invited to the third expert meeting to assist in the translation. He criticized that the project was 'regional', focusing too much on trivial differences among Asian states while ignoring potential users in the rest of the world and their concerns.[20] Wiseman's observation reflects the shaky basis of trust among these experts, whose nationalistic sentiments were readily aroused during the discussions. Even so, when Choi formed a task force team (TFT) that had fewer participants and concentrated more on the actual job, national differences were obscured by expressions of practical concern.

Aiming to construct a readable standard, the working language in the TFT meetings was not any single Asian language or English but, rather, a 'Creole' convenient for discussion. The presentation slides, for example, were in Chinese characters, which were from the classic texts and everyone was able to read. The discussion was carried on in either English or the local languages, with translations by interpreters. Some experts spoke two Asian languages and some communicated in English, but for crucial discrepancies they often demonstrated with their bodies – a language more universal even than English. Having a clear sense that the standard would be composed in English, the TFT was aware that a consensus of bodyscape had to be reached first and that its linguistic expression would be the final step toward the making of the standard.

Each point revealed different difficulties in the making of such consensus.[21] Some of the discrepancies are quite striking, given their wide popularity in research and practice. ST36, for example, is perhaps the most important point for promoting general wellness. The traditional approach to this point requires experience and skill to identify 'the anterior crest of the tibia', as written in the classics, in order to find this point one 'finger-breadth from it'. Even so, in the TFT meeting this was, surprisingly, one of the points for which it was hard to set a standard. Relying on the TFT's working motto that the standard need not be too bounded by 'either classics or anatomy', by 'clinical experience' or by 'national pride', the final result of the location of ST36 has nothing to do with bodily landmarks; the new standard indicates a point 'on the anterior aspect of the leg, on the line connecting ST35 with ST41, 3 B[one]-cun inferior to ST35' (WHO, 2008: 64).

In addition to those that just needed new descriptions, the most difficult points for setting standards were those that have distinctly different locations in each medical tradition. At the beginning of the TFT meetings Seung-hoon Choi insisted that no alternative locations would be allowed in the standard. However, this rule was broken as the meeting proceeded. For instance, in the traditional approach the location of GB30 is different in Japan from its location in the PRC and Korea (using the landmark of the greater trochanter, Japanese practitioners search for this point at its front, while their Chinese and Korean colleagues search for it at its rear). There was no way to find a common ground for this discrepancy, so alternative locations were inevitable. Even so, as can be read in the final standard, this contrast reads much more benignly as a result of the use of anatomical descriptions.[22]

In contrast to the case of GB30, the standard intends to make differences in the case of some points whose alternative locations are extremely close. For example, the two locations of PC9 are both at the edge of the nail on the middle finger, but the meanings behind these locations in meridian theory are so different that they cannot be reduced to one location. This principle also applied to GV26, where the distance between its two locations was only one sixth of the philtrum midline, meaning less than 0.5cm. In the end, six points in total had to have alternative locations noted in the standard.[23]

For outsiders these discrepancies seem ridiculous, as even professionals cannot exactly identify these points on the body. Even so, if we consider this standard seriously as a literary work it makes perfect sense to make such alternatives a part of it. Deviating from the rise of modern science in which representation is central and determinant, the standardization of acupuncture points should be understood as a translingual practice detached from either the body or its illustrative representation. If we read this bodyscape-named 'standard' carefully, we find that the standard is a dictionary-like narrative that contains descriptions of each point's literary/bodily location, like the glossary constructed in the 1980s. Alternative locations of points, just like linguistic variations in a dictionary, are listed, but explanations for the alternatives are missing. The terms used to compose this standard are mixed. Some are very ordinary and traditional, such as 'the tip of the nose'. However, for most points complicated anatomical terms are introduced which are difficult to read and follow.

Illustrations in the standard are accessory. Providing body shape and related bodily marks, such as bones, muscles and neighbouring points, they are to a degree more accessible for readers, but they fail to stand alone in making the invisible acupuncture points 'visible'. In fact, the leading expert of the Chinese delegation, Longxiang Huang, has commented that acupuncture points have to be approached from the body's surface but are not located there (Huang, 2005). Therefore, illustrations that contain only this kind of information are not useful. From a philosophical point of view, Huang's notion nicely reveals the techno-politics that can be seen in the standard. The general approach to the standardization of acupuncture points is literary rather than illustrative.

The way to interpret the standard, as Sergio Sismondo and Nicholas Chrisman (2001) would suggest, has to be like that of reading a map. The terms or illustrations are not used to clarify the location of these points on the body; instead, they are designed to achieve a certain obscurity and complexity that prevents readers from making a simple bodily correspondence.

Conclusion: mobile and translatable bodyscape and global health

Let me conclude this chapter with two contrasting pictures regarding the future of acupuncture. In 2010 the founder of Barefoot Acupuncturists, Dr Walter Fischer, shared his vision of global health with acupuncture (Team YS, 2010). Barefoot Acupuncturists, Fischer envisioned, would put effort into 'building up autonomous structures, giving acupuncture training in villages and slums'; with enthusiasm, he asserted, 'it can be achieved and we are sure that it will make the world a slightly better place'.

Leading a team in the research of TCM classics, the director of Horst-Görtz-Stiftungsinstitut für Theorie, Geschichte und Ethik Chinesischer Lebenswissenschaften, Paul Unschuld, emphasized his worries about the future of TCM, including the most distinctive acupuncture, in the 17th International Conference of Oriental Medicine, held in Taipei in November 2014. He noted that biomedicine would replace the theoretical foundation of TCM and make it merely a branch among other biomedical fields. Apparently, standardized acupuncture, by using anatomical terms, can be considered as one step in this direction.

Returning to our case, how do we assess the action taken to make acupuncture standardized? In October 2006, in Tsukuba, Japan, the WHO WPRO held a formal meeting on the standardization of acupuncture points. In addition to those from the PRC, Japan and Korea, experts from Australia, Singapore, Vietnam, Mongolia, the UK and the US joined the discussion, confirming decisions made in the expert meeting and discussing the six points at the centre of the controversy. No huge objection was made. One year from then was the final TFT meeting, where illustrations were finalized before the formal presentation of the standard in May 2008. As Seung-hoon Choi commented in the ceremony celebrating six years of hard work on it, 'At the moment when acupuncture locations are unified on the global level, ... we are the history makers in this field; the victory belongs to us' (Choi, 2008: 5).

It is indeed a progress; however, as this chapter has argued, the achievement has to be evaluated according to the techno-politics of the bodyscape. As this chapter has revealed, in the making of this standard some things have been singled out, while others are missing. Points replaced meridians, to appear as the main body of the text; and illustrations are considered to be accessories to their textual expressions. From this viewpoint, what is at stake in such a text may be neither whether it will provide accessibility for more students in the world, nor whether it will destroy the authenticity of this healing art but, rather, the following: how on Earth can this standard be followed?

From a philosophical perspective, perhaps standardized acupuncture does not matter much to those who practise it. As Ludwig Wittgenstein argued in *Philosophical Investigations* (1958 [1953]), more rules do not guarantee more precise explanations; they still leave doubts by those who use them (aphorism 85). For practitioners, it is fair to say that acupuncture points, being standardized and 'pinned down' on the body, are signposts: they will never be able to offer exact guidance for treatment. Nonetheless, Wittgenstein also discussed how people follow unperfected rules (aphorism 198). In the case of acupuncture, the standard will not change everything at once; regular ways of using and receiving it can emerge among acupuncture masters, disciples and patients who receive such therapeutic interventions.

What is equally important between the lines of this standard is an emerging bodyscape that is ready to invite new modes of interpretation/dispute. Upon its formal release the standard of acupuncture point locations soon became the subject of a political battle over 'whose standard was adopted as the global standard'. Angry at the announcement by the Korean Association of Acupuncture that the standard is a victory of Korea because more than 99% of points in it follow the Korean standard, the PRC insisted that 359 of the 361 points are similar to the Chinese standard. While Japan emphasizes its contribution to the standard, Taiwan, the outsider of the discussion, sent corrections directly to the WHO headquarters in order to seek visibility (Lin et al., 2011). Departing from a geopolitical reading of the standard, this chapter has suggested that, from the manner of its making, it should instead be read both politically and scientifically.

Londa Schiebinger (1993) successfully demonstrated the politics of naming as embedded in placing mammals in the taxonomy of species. In the case of acupuncture, I would like to suggest that the politics is more cartographic. As this chapter insists, it is the bodyscape, the 'map' in a deflationary sense, not the politics about it, that is at stake in this debate. To make a readable standard for the makers and projected users, the bodyscape has to be translated from classical texts and its different interpretations are introduced by people. The techno-politics, as I argue repeatedly, is embedded in the making of such a standard.

And the techno-politics does not end with the establishment of the standard. It will travel as 'immutable mobiles', to borrow Bruno Latour's notion, which will facilitate the circulation of acupuncture in classrooms, clinics, research laboratories and international meetings in the world via 'visual consistency'. Meanwhile, as a textual presentation of the bodyscape, this standard has been made readable, presentable, combinable and also translatable. It is in this sense that acupuncture in its modern form demonstrates an epistemic turn to global health.

Also following Latour's (1991) provocative notion which claims that 'we have never been modern', perhaps we should ask ourselves, as well as those who believe that the standards of acupuncture will lead to the modernization of this healing art and age-old bodily technique, a simple question: have we ever gotten the point?

Notes

1 James Reston, one of Nixon's accompanying journalists, had an acute appendicitis attack. Chinese physicians performed an emergency operation on Reston and afterward used acupuncture to ease his pain. See Prensky (1995).
2 See the official website of Barefoot Acupuncturists, www.barefootacupuncturists.com/theprojest.htm (accessed 8 February 2016).
3 I have argued elsewhere the necessity of reassessing Needham's legacy as both a Sibologist and a serious scientist in pursuing science that is universal (Kuo, 2019).
4 An excellent comparison is given by sociologist Deborah Lupton, who in her classic work (1994) pointed out that, even among Western societies,

where biomedicine dominates, the ways in which to conceive an illness and the body in therapeutic contexts vary.
5 For example, in its illustration (127), *L'Acuponcture Chinoise* wrongly spells GB1 (tungtsuliao) as tungtsuchao because the last character '髎' (liao) looks like '膠' (chao).
6 For example, after passing ST5 (大迎), some numbering systems indicate a upward qi go through the point '頰車" (ST6), while some systems number the point that succeeds ST5 '人迎' (ST9), indicating that the upward line to the top of head is a branch of Stomach meridian.
7 See, for example, 'Acupuncture to get heritage designation', *Chinadaily*, 14 September 2010, www.chinadaily.com.cn/imqq/china/2010-09/14/content_11300649.htm (accessed 8 February 2016).
8 These scientists include (in the order of the years of their main research findings): Yoshio Nagahama (長濱善夫, 1950), Rokuro Fujita (藤田六郎, 1952), Jean, F. Borsarello (1970), Tong Wang (汪桐, 1972), Zhaowei Meng (孟昭威, 1978), Baozhen Zhang (張保真, 1980), Hungary Eore (1984), Haozan Xie (謝浩然, 1984), Claude Darras and *Pierre De Vernejou (1985) and* Jacques-Emile Henri Niboyet (1985).
9 Nakatani found 370 points, 9 points more than recorded in classics of acupuncture.
10 In retrospect, the first world conference on acupuncture and moxibustion was held in Japan in 1965. The second was held in Paris in May 1969, the third in Seoul in September 1973, the fourth in Las Vegas of Nevada, the fifth in Tokyo in October 1977.
11 To take the world conferences on acupuncture and moxibustion as an example, before the PRC established its own international organization, the World Federation of Acupuncture Societies (WFAS), in 1987, the visibility of Chinese delegates increased. The seventh world conference on acupuncture and moxibustion, held in Kuala Lumpur in 1978, had two papers from PRC representatives, one of which was on the nomenclature of acupuncture points. The eighth, held in 1983, had nine delegates from the PRC.
12 The following account of the early attempts to create a standard for acupuncture is based on Kiichiro Tsutani's report after completing his service at WHO-WPRO (Tsutani, 1992a and 1992b).
13 Personal communication with Kiichiro Tsutani in connection with the translation from Japanese to Chinese in 2012 of his eventually unpublished manuscript titled 'Making Harmonies among East Asian Medicines'.
14 In fact, among the states that recognize acupuncture as a legal practice, Taiwan is the only one in which traditional Chinese characters are still

Acupuncture and the techno-politics of bodyscape   149

used as an official language. Even so, for political reasons it is not formally invited to these projects.

15 Interview with Seung-hoon Choi at Korean Institute of Oriental Medicine, 16 February 2014.
16 The so-called 'bone-cun' measurement system. Rather than taking a fixed length as the unit of measurement, the length of each unit in this system varies, depending on the proportion of skeleton by which the *acupuncture* points on that part of the body are located.
17 In addition to Choi from the WPRO, the experts included Xuetai Wang (王雪苔), Longxian Huang (黄龙祥), Zhigao Jin (晋志高) and Ding Li (李鼎) from the PRC, Sung Gil Kang (姜成吉), Yong Suk Kim (金容奭) and Hye Jung Lee (李惠貞) from Korea and Shuichi Katai (形井秀一), Shuji Shinohara (篠原昭二), Kenji Kobayashi (小林健二), Hisatsugu Urayama (浦山久嗣) and Kika Urayama (浦山きか, as Chinese interpreter) from Japan.
18 In contrast to this approach, one expert proposed the concept of 'basic points' which function as the 'hub' for other points which can be reached through these points. However, this proposal failed to win approval in the meeting.
19 For example, the GB31(風市) point is traditionally approached as follows: if the patient is standing erect with his/her hands close to the sides, the point is where the tip of the middle finger touches. I will include more discussion on this point in a longer version of this chapter.
20 Interview with Nigel Wiseman, Taipei, 25 February 2014.
21 The fourth informal meeting of the Standard of Acupuncture Point Location group in 2005 confirmed three types of discrepancies. The first type consisted of the eighteen points that have discrepancies in location, such as LI20 (迎香), ST30 (氣衝), SP11 (箕門), SP12 (衝門), PC8 (勞宮), PC9 (中衝), SJ18 (瘈脈), GB9 (天衝), GB10 (浮白), GB19 (腦空), LR4 (中封), LR5 (蠡溝), LR6 (中都), LR7 (膝関), GV26 (水溝), BL6 (承光), BL7 (通天) and BL9 (玉枕). The second type consisted of those that have the same location but different expressions for this location, such as LU3 (天府), LU4 (俠白), ST4 (地倉), LI7 (温溜), KI1 (湧泉), GB4 (頷厭), SJ19 (顱息), GB16 (目窗), GB17 (正營), GB30 (環跳), GB31 (風市), GB32 (中瀆), LR9 (陰包), LR10 (足五里), LR11 (陰廉) and LR12 (急脈). The third type of discrepancy occurred in twenty-four points where primary consensus had been reached but later the PRC asked for more discussion, including LI12 (肘髎), ST36 (足三里), ST37 (上巨虛), ST38 (條口), ST39 (下巨虛), ST41 (解溪), ST42 (衝陽), BL1 (睛明), BL39 (委陽), KI9 (築賓), TE9 (四瀆), TE15 (天髎), TE16 (天牖), GB7 (曲鬢), GB21 (肩井), GB23 (輒筋), GB25 (京門), GB27 (五樞), GB28

(維道), LR3 (太衝), CV21 (璇璣), SI19 (聽宮), TE12 (消濼) and TE13 (臑會).

22 The standard location of GB30 (環跳) reads as follows: 'In the buttock region, at the junction of the lateral one third and medical two thirds of the line connecting the prominence of the greater trochanter with the sacral hiatus. Remarks: Alternative location for GB30 – In the buttock region, at the junction of the lateral one third and medical two thirds of the distance between the prominence of the greater trochanter and anterior iliac spine' (WHO, 2008: 180).

23 For these points, the experts voted to decide which location would be mentioned in the text, with the other location being mentioned in the remarks.

References

Candelise, Lucia (2008) *La médecine chinoise dans la pratique médicale en France et en Italie, de 1930 à nos jours. Représentations, réception, tentatives d'intégration* (Chinese Medicines, in Medical Practice in France and Italy, from 1930 to today. Representations, Reception, Attempts of Appropriation), Ph.D. dissertation, Histoire et Civilisations et Anthropologie culturelle, EHESS, CECMC, UMR 8173 Chine Corée Japon, Paris.

Choi, Seung-hoon (崔昇勳) (2008) 'WHO hyojun keiketubuishupan kinenkouen ni yosete' (WHO 標準経穴部位出版紀念講演によせて, Memorial remarks on the publication of *WHO Standard Acupuncture Point Locations in the Western Pacific Region*). Pamphlet of WHO/WPRO hyojun keiketubui kousikipan hakan kinen kouenkai. Kyoto, 4–5.

Duden, Barbara (1991) *The Woman Beneath the Skin: A Doctor's Patients in Eighteenth-Century Germany*. Cambridge, MA: Harvard University Press.

Furth, Charlotte (2011) 'The AMS/Paterson lecture: Becoming alternative? Modern transformations of Chinese medicine in China and in the United States', *Canadian Bulletin of Medical History / Bulletin canadien d'histoire de la medicine* 28 (1), 5–41.

Harley, John Brian (1988) 'Maps, knowledge and power', in *The Iconography of Landscape: Essays on the Symbolic Representation, Design, and Use of Past Environments*, ed. D. Cosgrove and S. Daniels (pp. 277–312). Cambridge: Cambridge University Press.

Hsu, Elisabeth (1999) *The Transmission of Chinese Medicine*. Cambridge: Cambridge University Press.

Huang, Longxiang (黄龙祥) (2005) 'Dongjing guoli bowuguan zhenjiu tongjen yenjiu de tupou yu fansi" (东京国立博物馆针灸铜人研究的突破与反思, Reflections and breakthroughs on the research of bronze acupuncture figure

at Tokyo National Museum). *Ziran kexueshi yenjiu* (Studies the History of Natural Sciences) 24 (1), 1–12.
Knorr-Cetina, Karin and Klaus Amann (1990) 'Image dissection in natural scientific inquiry', *Science, Technology, & Human Values* 15 (3), 259–283.
Kuo, Wen-Hua (2019) 'An ecumenical medicine yet to come: reflections on Needham on Medicine', *Isis* 110 (1), 116–121.
Kuriyama, Shigehisa (1999) *The Expressiveness of the Body and the Divergence of Greek and Chinese Medicine*. New York: Zone books.
Laqueur, Thomas (1992) *Making Sex: Body and Gender from the Greeks to Freud*. Cambridge, MA: Harvard University Press.
Latour, Bruno (1986) 'Visualisation and cognition: drawing things together', in special issue of in *Knowledge and Society: Studies in the Sociology of Culture Past and Present* (edited by H. Kuklick), 6, 1–40. Greenwich, CT: Jai Press.
Latour, Bruno (1991) *We Have Never Been Modern*. Translated by Catherine Porter. Cambridge, MA: Harvard University Press.
Lei, S. H. (2014) *Neither Donkey nor Horse: Medicine in the Struggle over China's Modernity*. Chicago: University of Chicago Press.
Lin, Jaung-Geng (林昭庚), Yu-Chen Lee (李育臣), Ya-Ting Wu (吳雅婷), Yi-Hung Chen (陳易宏) (2011) 'due xitaipingyangdichu WHO biaojunzhenjiuxueweizhixiudingjianyi'(對《西太平洋地區WHO標準針灸穴位》之修訂建議, A suggestion to revise the *WHO Standard Acupuncture Point Locations in the Western Pacific Region*), *Taiwan Zhongyi Yixue Zhazhi* (台灣中醫醫學雜誌) 10 (3), 1–10.
Liu, Lydia H. (1995) *Translingual Practice: Literature, National Culture, and Translated Modernity—China, 1900–1937*. Stanford, CA: Stanford University Press.
Lock, Margaret (1993) *Encounters with Aging: Mythologies of Menopause in Japan and North America*. Berkeley: University of California Press.
Lock, Margaret (2002) *Twice Dead: Organ Transplants and the Reinvention of Death*. Berkeley: University of California Press.
Lock, Margaret and Vinh-Kim Nguyen (2010) *An Anthropology of Biomedicine*. Oxford: Wiley-Blackwell.
Lock, Stephen, John M. Last and George Dunea (eds) (2001) *The Oxford Illustrated Companion to Medicine* (3rd edn). Oxford: Oxford University Press.
Lu, Gwei-Djen and Joseph Needham (2002 [1980]) *Celestial Lancets: A History and Rationale of Acupuncture and Moxa*. London: Routledge.
Lupton, Deborah (1994) *Medicine as Culture: Illness, Disease, and the Body in Western Societies*. London: Sage.
Ma, Eunjeong and Michael Lynch (2014) 'Constructing the East–West boundary: the contested place of a modern imaging technology in South Korea's dual medical system', *Science, Technology, & Human Values* 39 (5), 639–665.

Needham, Joseph (1969) *The Grand Titration: Science and Society in East and West*. London: Allen & Unwin.
Prensky, William (1995) 'Reston Helped Open a Door to Acupuncture', *New York Times*, 14 December, A30.
Pritzker, Sonya E. (2014) 'Standardization and its discontents: translation, tension, and the life of language in contemporary Chinese medicine', *East Asian Science, Technology and Society: an International Journal* 8 (1), 25–42.
Rubach, Axel (2001 [1995]) *Principles of Ear Acupuncture: Microsystem of the Auricle*. New York: Thieme.
Scheid, Volker (2002) *Chinese Medicine in Contemporary China: Plurality and Synthesis*. Durham, NC: Duke University Press.
Scheid, Volker and Hugh MacPherson (eds) (2012) *Integrating East Asian Medicine into Contemporary Healthcare*. London: Churchill Livingstone.
Schiebinger, Londa (1993) 'Why mammals are called mammals: gender politics in eighteenth-century natural history', *The American Historical Review* 98 (2), 382–411.
Shapin, Steven and Simon Schaffer (1985) *Leviathan and the Air-Pump: Hobbes, Boyle, and the Experimental Life*. Princeton, NJ: Princeton University Press.
Sismondo, Sergio and Nicholas Chrisman (2001) 'Deflationary metaphysics and the natures of maps', *Proceedings of the Philosophy of Science Association 2001* 3, S38–S49.
Team YS (2010) 'Dr. Walter Fischer, Barefoot Acupuncturists, Dharavi, Mumbai', Your Story, http://yourstory.com/2010/12/dr-walter-fischer-barefoot-acupuncturists-dharavi-mumbai/ (accessed 8 February 2016).
Tsutani, Kiichiro (津谷喜一郎) (1992a) 'Sekaikyotu no shinkyugo wo nezashite – kogoku de no sinyogo no ugoki (sono ichi)' (世界共通の鍼灸語をねざして-各国での鍼用語の動き (その1), Have a universally communicable language on acupuncture deeply rooted: the national situations of acupuncture languages I). *Gendai Toyo Yigaku* (現代東洋醫學) 12 (4), 39–44.
Tsutani, Kiichiro (津谷喜一郎) (1992b) 'Sekaikyotu no shinkyugo wo nezashite – kogoku de no sinyogo no ugoki (sono ichi)' (世界共通の鍼灸語をねざして-各国での鍼用語の動き (その2), Have a universally communicable language on acupuncture deeply rooted: the national situations of acupuncture languages II), *Gendai Toyo Yigaku* (現代東洋醫學) 13 (1), 45–58.
Vertesi, Janet (2008) 'The London Underground map and users' representations of urban space', *Social Studies of Science* 38 (1), 7–33.
Wang, Deshen (王德深) (1987) 'A proposal for the international standardization of acupuncture point names', in *Zhenjiuxueming guojibiaozhunhua shouce* (針灸穴名國際標準化手冊, Manual of international standardization of acupuncture point names) (pp. 10–23). Taichung: weishen chupanshe.

Wittgenstein, Ludwig (1958 [1953]) *Philosophical Investigations: The English text of the third edition*, translated by G. E. M. Anscombe. London: Basil Blackwell & Mott Ltd.

WHO (2008) *WHO Standard Acupuncture Point Locations in the Western Pacific Region*. Manila: WHO Regional Office for the Western Pacific.

Zhan, Mei (2009) *Other-Worldly: Making Chinese Medicine through Transnational Frames*. Durham, NC: Duke University Press.

Zhang, Weibo (波) (2012) *Jinluo yu jiankang* (经络与健康, Meridians and health). Beijing: Renmin weishen chupanshe.

7

Finding the global in the local: constructing population in the search for disease genes

Steve Sturdy

Introduction

Since the birth of genetics in the early twentieth century geneticists have been keen to understand what their science can say about how humans differ from one another, including how they differ from one part of the globe to another. Since the early 1990s there has been a notable surge in initiatives aiming to describe and analyse the genetic make-up of people living outside Europe and North America. Some of these initiatives profess a primarily anthropological orientation, aiming to capture and document as much as possible of the sheer diversity of human genetic constitutions: the Human Genome Diversity Project and National Geographic's Genographic Project are cases in point. Other initiatives – often framed in terms of documenting genetic 'variation' rather than 'diversity' – claim a more practical orientation towards identifying gene variants of medical significance: the International Haplotype Mapping (HapMap) Project and the African Genome Variation Project exemplify this latter approach to human genetics. In explaining the medical value of such work, advocates commonly state that it will generate genetic information that will help to combat illness and foster health in the countries under study. Thus the International HapMap Project is framed in terms of the 'need to be inclusive in the populations that we study to maximize the chance that all people will eventually benefit from this international research effort' (NIH News Advisory, 2002); while the African Genome Variation Project is presented as a step towards 'provid[ing] a comprehensive resource for medical genomic studies in Africa' (Gurdasani et al., 2015: 331).

In this chapter I look beyond such professions of intent to examine a broader set of drivers that have structured the global expansion of genomic research and that skew how its findings are used. I show how recent initiatives to document the genetic constitution of people living in the world's poorer regions have actually grown out of, and serve the purposes of, efforts to identify genetic factors which influence the health of people living predominantly in the global North. This is perhaps unsurprising. For one thing, most research into the genetics of disease and ill health has been conducted by researchers based in the wealthiest countries of Europe and North America. For another, such research is to a significant extent driven by commercial interests, in the hope of profiting financially from any resulting medical innovations; consequently, research has tended to focus on understanding the ailments affecting those sections of the world's population that are most likely to be able to afford such innovations. In which case, why the recent turn to study the genomes of people living outside these rich regions? This chapter sets out to answer this question through a historical study of the changing aims and methodologies of medical genetics and human population genetics, and their recent convergence around new approaches to identifying genetic causes of ill health and disease.

Based on a close reading of medical genetics research literature, I show how, between the 1980s and the early 2000s, the focus of that research shifted from rare single-gene disorders to the genetics of common complex disorders such as heart disease and diabetes. I show how that shift in focus involved a shift in methodology: from studying the hereditary transmission of disease within families, to searching for correlations between genes and disease in populations. In particular, I show how a new approach to characterizing and analysing genetic populations came to be articulated in the course of this methodological turn. This new approach arose from the hybridization of two different and longer-established ways of thinking about populations. On the one hand, it drew on mainstream epidemiological ideas of populations as artificial constructs, created and defined for the purposes of research itself. And on the other hand, it drew on ideas inherited from older approaches to human population genetics which supposed that distinct genetic populations, far from being constructed by researchers, actually exist in nature and are simply characterized and differentiated through the use of appropriate research methods. I argue that the adoption of this novel approach to populations as a basis for identifying genetic causes of common disorders was one of the principal drivers, in the 1990s, for the surge of interest in the genetics of people living outside the global North. Specifically, as we shall see, knowledge of particular genotypes that occur with different frequency in different parts of the world was deemed necessary so as to control for the confounding effects of so-called 'population structure' in the search for correlations between diseases and genes. In practice, this knowledge has overwhelmingly been used to facilitate research into disease–gene correlations among white Europeans and North Americans. As a result, the net effect of the globalization of genetic research has not been to reduce global inequalities in research into disease, its causes and treatment, but, if anything, to exacerbate them.

Populations and disease genes in the 1950s to 1970s

During the immediate post-war years research into human population genetics and research into genetic factors in human disease tended to diverge in their aims and methods. Consider first the research aimed at identifying genetic causes of disease. Such work focused primarily on single-gene disorders. These are mostly rare conditions, such as Huntington's disease or phenylketonuria, in which individuals possessing either one or more usually two variant copies (depending on the condition) of a particular gene will usually develop, sooner or later, the phenotypic signs of that condition. In such disorders researchers can trace transmission of the relevant genetic variants through successive generations of a family using the theoretical schema of Mendelian genetics. Family pedigrees accordingly served as the principal objects of research for medical geneticists interested in identifying and tracking such disorders, and remained so during the 1960s and 1970s, with researchers often devoting considerable effort to seeking out and cultivating affected families (see, inter alia, Comfort, 2012: 97–129; Gaudillière, 2000; Lindee, 2005; Nukaga, 2002).

As well as following the inheritance of genetic disorders from one generation to the next, medical geneticists were also keen to map the location of the causal gene variants onto the human chromosomes. Gene-mapping techniques had been developed from the 1920s by geneticists working in the laboratory with experimental animals and plants. These techniques involved observing a phenomenon known as linkage. According to classical Mendelian genetics, in the course of sexual reproduction the alleles of any one gene will normally be distributed among members of the next generation quite independently of the alleles of any other gene. However, if two genes happen to be situated close together on the same chromosome their alleles will tend to be inherited together in a non-random fashion; in such cases, the genes are said to display linkage. The greater the tendency for alleles to be inherited together, the closer the linkage, and the closer together the relevant genes are assumed to be situated on the chromosome. By conducting controlled mutation and breeding experiments and observing multiple Mendelian traits, by the early post-war years geneticists had been able to construct genetic linkage maps of a range of organisms from the fruit fly *Drosophila* to maize and laboratory mice (Kohler, 1994; Rheinberger and Gaudillière, 2004).

Linkage mapping in experimental organisms played an important role in the development of genetics as a scientific discipline during the first half of the twentieth century. For medical geneticists it also offered a possible route to more practical benefits. If a genetic disorder could be shown to be linked to a more easily observable trait, the presence of that trait might serve as a diagnostic marker, enabling clinical geneticists to identify the disease before the onset of symptoms or to identify carriers who would not themselves develop the disease but could pass on the offending genetic variant to their offspring. Humans did not lend themselves well to available methods of genetic linkage mapping, however. For one thing, humans are not generally regarded as appropriate subjects for systematic breeding experiments. For another, humans are a young species in evolutionary terms and so are less genetically diverse than many other organisms. Consequently, they exhibit relatively few of the kinds of Mendelian traits that can be followed from one generation to the next. Given the paucity of such traits, such genetic linkage maps as were constructed up to the late 1970s contained relatively few genes, including no more than a handful of genetic disorders, while the degrees of linkage remained too tenuous to be of diagnostic or predictive value (Harper, 2008: 194–212).

While medical geneticists concentrated on families in their search for disease genes, human population geneticists pursued a rather different set of concerns during the post-war decades. Their principal aim was to elucidate the history and dynamics of human evolution – an enterprise which they conducted in sometimes fractious dialogue with physical anthropologists (Smocovitis, 2012). Beginning in the nineteenth century, studies of human evolution initially focused on efforts to characterize distinct races of humanity and to chart the hierarchical relationships between them. The anthropological and anthropometric techniques employed for this purpose were augmented during the first half of the twentieth century by new genetic methods of defining and differentiating populations, in particular by observing differences in the frequency of certain common genotypes. In particular, the realization that the ABO system of blood groups followed a simple pattern of genetic determination paved the way to large-scale population surveys of the distribution of different genotypes, made possible by the ease of collecting, storing, transporting and serotyping blood samples (Gannet and Griesemer, 2004; Marks, 2012). The post-war years saw further expansion in both the scale and geographical scope of such surveys, as well as the identification of additional serological markers of genetic difference (Bangham, 2014; Radin, 2014).

At the same time, dominant views about the nature of human evolutionary relationships were shifting as anthropologists and geneticists alike sought to cast off earlier, overtly racist assumptions about human difference. By the 1960s concerns to identify distinct racial types had largely given way to a more dynamic and relativistic understanding of human population. Earlier race theorists had posited that races constituted discrete geographically or reproductively separate populations. By contrast, post-war population geneticists were increasingly inclined to envisage a single, continuous global population connected by constant migration and interbreeding and structured not by discrete boundaries but by continuous variation in gene frequency from one part of the world to another. Consequently, they argued, biology could provide no basis for essentialist ideas of race. However, disagreements remained over whether this shift in thinking meant that it no longer made sense to talk about biological races at all. Some post-war human geneticists argued that it was still possible to discern distinct human populations separated by cultural as well as geographical barriers. Even if the boundaries between those populations were blurred and porous, they still placed enough restrictions in the way of genetic exchange, and the populations they demarcated were still sufficiently different in their genetic make-up, to constitute distinct biological races. Others adopted a more pragmatic viewpoint. Discrete populations might not exist in reality, they argued. But for purposes of genetic research into human difference it was useful to behave as if they did, using geographical or other criteria to demarcate populations to sample and study. As a number of historians have observed, such research commonly drew on ethnic and other markers of population difference. In so doing it tended to reintroduce, albeit implicitly, older assumptions about race into the identification of populations for purposes of human genetic research. At the same time, that research itself tended to naturalize and reify those assumptions by showing that, in many cases, genetic differences could indeed be found between the populations so defined. While the precise relationship of these genetic differences to other forms of racial, ethnic or geographical difference continued to be debated, the circular reasoning underlying much of that research went largely unremarked, thereby helping to sediment assumptions that racial and ethnic differences are at least partly rooted in biology (see, inter alia, Bangham, 2015; Gannet, 2001, 2003; Gannet and Griesemer 2004; Gormley, 2009; Lipphardt, 2014; Marks, 2012; Reardon, 2004, 2005; Smocovitis, 2012).

On the whole, this line of research into population genetics offered little of practical interest to medical geneticists, at least at that time. Medical geneticists did sometimes take an ambivalent interest in the kinds of large-scale population surveys of variation in gene frequency that flourished in the post-war decades (de Chadarevian, 2014) – chiefly in the hope that they would provide insight into hereditary influences on susceptibility to infectious diseases and common disorders such as heart disease, as well as rare single-gene disorders. However, while such research certainly provided new epidemiological information about variability in disease incidence, it was less informative about supposed genetic determinants of that variation. Even where such research helped to throw new epidemiological light on the incidence of rare genetic disorders those findings were rarely of much practical benefit to medical geneticists. The observation that gene variants associated with sickle cell disease appeared to confer a selective advantage on people living in malarial regions of the world, for instance, provided population geneticists with a neat example of how evolutionary theory could be applied to humans. For medical geneticists, meanwhile, the same findings helped to direct diagnostic attention in ways that often reflected racial assumptions about predisposition to disease (Wailoo and Pemberton, 2008). More generally, evidence of population-based variation in disease incidence proved largely unpersuasive as an argument for genetic causation: unless researchers could demonstrate clear Mendelian patterns of inheritance, they found it difficult to argue that increased incidence was due to genetic rather than environmental causes, as was evident for instance in the case of familial cancers (Cantor, 2006; Necochea, 2007). Consequently, despite the growth in research into population genetics during the 1960s and 1970s, medical geneticists continued to focus their attention on families rather than populations.

However, there was one important exception to this generalization. One key site where the interests of population geneticists and medical geneticists came into productive dialogue with one another was in relation to so-called 'population isolates'. Population geneticists had coined this term to denote specific populations which they considered to have been reproductively isolated, be it for geographical or cultural reasons, from the larger human gene pool. Groups identified as population isolates were typically quite small in size, although they included some larger groups such as the Finns and the Basques. They were also considered to be atypical in a world elsewhere dominated by movement and interbreeding. And that atypicality made them uniquely valuable. Human geneticists regarded population isolates as relics from older periods of population history, biologically untouched by more recent flows of people and genes that had shaped present-day populations. As such, they were seen to offer unique insight into human evolution. But they were also seen to be at risk. With the growing speed and reach of modern population movements, small population isolates were increasingly vulnerable to out-breeding, dilution and, ultimately, dissolution. Consequently, population geneticists were anxious to sample and characterize such isolates before they were lost to the homogenizing flood of modernity, and the 1960s and 1970s saw a number of gene-hunting expeditions launched, particularly to sample such supposedly 'primitive' peoples as the Yanomami whose isolation was assumed to stretch back furthest in evolutionary time (Lindee, 2003; Lipphardt, 2012, 2014).

Medical geneticists, too, were keen to study population isolates – although for rather different reasons than population geneticists. For medical geneticists, population isolates represented unusually fertile ground on which to hunt for rare genetic diseases. Often descended from small groups of founders, with high rates of in-breeding and consanguinity, population isolates were typically judged to possess relatively low genetic diversity. Consequently, while such populations would likely harbour fewer genetic disorders, any disorders that did occur would do so with far higher frequency than in a larger, more heterogeneous population, recurring repeatedly in the pedigrees of densely interrelated families. Medical geneticists were therefore keen to work with population isolates as a means of identifying disorders which they would find much harder spot elsewhere. Unlike population geneticists, however, they tended to be less concerned with evolutionary 'primitiveness' than by accessibility and the availability of well-validated family histories. Consequently, medical geneticists were as likely to conduct their research among culturally defined 'isolates' living in Europe and North America, such as Ashkenazi Jews and the Pennsylvania Amish, as among more geographically remote populations (Lindee, 2005: 58–89, 156–186; Wailoo and Pemberton, 2008; Widmer, 2014).

This shared interest in population isolates was one of the few places where ideas from population genetics intersected directly with the medical geneticists' efforts to identify disease genes. Overall, work in human population genetics and research into genetic causes of human disease were notable as much for the extent to which they tended to diverge, both theoretically and methodologically, as for their occasional overlaps. Where population geneticists focused on statistical observations of the frequency of common variants within freely interbreeding populations, medical geneticists were concerned primarily with tracing individual occurrences of rare genetic variants within families. This divergence would become more marked during the 1980s as medical geneticists adopted new techniques from molecular genetics that enabled them to focus ever more clearly on families rather than other kinds of human grouping.

Family studies and molecular mapping

As we have seen, the possibility of conducting genetic linkage studies in humans was severely constrained, up to the 1970s, by the paucity of common, phenotypically observable genetic variants. However, the development of new molecular biotechnologies during the 1970s made it possible to circumvent some of those constraints by identifying a growing number of variants which do not usually give rise to observable phenotypic differences but which can be identified in the laboratory using molecular biological techniques. These included so-called restriction fragment length polymorphisms (RFLPs) – specific combinations of nucleic acids that can occur at various points in the genome, which began to be identified in humans in significant numbers from the late 1970s; and later, from the early 1990s, microsatellite variants – repetitive sequences of nucleotides scattered through the genome, which vary in the number of repeats. Both RFLPs and microsatellite variants proved to be much commoner in humans than the kinds of phenotypically expressed gene variants that had previously been used for linkage studies. As such, they provided medical geneticists with a new and powerful set of techniques for studying linkage in humans, and ultimately for mapping conditions such as rare genetic disorders that could be shown to be linked to these genomic markers.

Medical geneticists first adopted the idea of using RFLP markers to study linkage to human disease genes in the late 1970s (Kan and Dozy, 1978; Solomon and Bodmer, 1979). The first steps in this direction were initiated by the Hereditary Disease Foundation (HDF), set up in 1968 by Dr Milton Wexler following his wife's diagnosis with Huntington's disease, with the aim of promoting research into Huntington's and other genetic conditions. In 1979 the HDF funded a group of geneticists to try to map the Huntington's disease gene using the new RFLP markers. The researcher worked first with an 'American family of reasonable size' identified through the National Research Roster for Huntington's Disease Patients and Families at Indiana University, and subsequently with what the researchers described as 'a unique community of interrelated Huntingdon's disease gene carriers living along the shores of Lake Maracaibo, Venezuela'. The researchers struck lucky. Employing a panel of only a dozen RFLP markers, in 1983 they were able to report the mapping of Huntington's disease to chromosome 4, and the identification of an RFLP marker of potential value in identifying individuals who carried the fatal genetic variant (Gusella et al., 1983; Nukaga, 2002: 53–57).

Meanwhile, in 1980 a group of American molecular biologists had proposed that a concerted programme of identifying RFLPs should be undertaken with the aim of constructing a linkage map of the whole human genome, in order to facilitate more systematic mapping of genes associated with hereditary diseases (Botstein et al., 1980). In 1984, as the work on Huntington's disease made clear the potential of such an approach, a group of researchers from the US and France agreed to set up an international collaboration, sharing biological materials and analytical skills with the aim of creating the first complete human linkage map. The Centre d'Etude du Polymorphisme Humain (CEPH), as this collaboration was called, drew on three sets of three-generation families. In France, over 100 families had been recruited during the 1970s to provide a tissue-type reference group for the French tissue transplantation services; ten of these families were subsequently brought into the CEPH. In the US, researchers at the Howard Hughes Medical Institute in Salt Lake City, including two of the authors of the original 1980 paper proposing the construction of an RFLP linkage map, recruited a group of Mormon families. Two large families from the ongoing Huntington's disease study in Venezuela were also added to the CEPH's reference panel. Cell lines and pedigree data from these families were distributed to an increasingly large network of researchers and the results of linkage experiments were shared among the collaborators (Dausset et al., 1990; Rabinow, 1999). Using these resources, the first genetic linkage map of the whole human genome, involving over 400 genomic markers, was published in 1987 (Donis-Keller et al., 1987).

By that time, RFLP linkage data from the CEPH were already being successfully used to demonstrate linkage in a variety of hereditary diseases. In 1985 a collaborative study of forty-three Canadian families with children affected by cystic fibrosis made use of the accumulating body of RFLP markers to report a linked marker on chromosome 7 (Knowlton et al., 1985; Tsui et al., 1985). Other conditions quickly followed, including chronic granulomatous disease, Duchenne muscular dystrophy and a rare genetic cancer called retinoblastoma. Clinical geneticists added the linked markers to the range of tools at their disposal for diagnosing and predicting these diseases. Detailed study of the inheritance of single-gene disorders through large pedigrees such as the Venezuelan Huntington's disease cohort in turn yielded additional markers that could be used to map other genes (Jones and Tansey, 2015, 33). By 1986 advocates of RFLP linkage mapping felt sufficiently confident to suggest that 'RFLPs can be found linked to any common human disease that shows simple Mendelian transmission and is caused by a single genetic locus' (Lander and Botstein, 1986: 49). Their confidence was further boosted during the early 1990s as researchers added microsatellite variants to their panels of RFLP markers, enabling them to produce even denser linkage maps of the human genome, while also streamlining the process of genotyping samples in the laboratory (Kaufmann, 2004; Kruglyak, 2008: 314; Weissenbach et al., 1992). By that time, molecular geneticists were not simply mapping the markers linked with hereditary diseases but also isolating, cloning and sequencing the genes themselves. Building on medical geneticists' well-established methods of studying inheritance within families, genomic linkage mapping had become a highly productive tool for researchers and clinicians working in the genetics of rare diseases.

Towards association studies

At the same time, researchers were becoming increasingly frustrated by the limitations of family studies. Such studies were effective for mapping the kinds of single-gene disorders which follow Mendelian patterns of transmission and segregation from one generation to the next. But Mendelian conditions are mostly rare, and attracted little medical interest beyond the specialism of medical genetics. With rapid developments in molecular biology yielding powerful new research tools, by the early 1990s scientists were growing increasingly ambitious to identify genetic determinants not just of Mendelian disorders but also of common disorders such as diabetes and heart disease.

It had long been known that elevated risk of developing some of the commonest health disorders often runs in families. Since the late 1950s a growing body of research using twin studies and other methods had provided geneticists with what they regarded as compelling evidence that a significant proportion of that elevated risk was hereditary rather than environmental in origin (Lindee, 2005, ch. 5). However, such conditions rarely displayed anything that could be identified as Mendelian patterns of inheritance; they occurred sporadically, albeit more frequently in certain families than in others – a fact that geneticists attributed to the involvement of multiple genes, each of which contributed to the probability of disease occurring but was insufficient on its own to make that occurrence a certainty. Researchers agreed that, given the sporadic occurrence of such conditions within affected families, family linkage methods were largely useless for mapping the predisposing genes (e.g. Lander and Botstein, 1986).

Confronted with these limitations, researchers began to consider other methods that they believed would be better suited to identifying the genetic factors involved in complex disorders. In place of the kind of one-to-one correspondences between genotype and disease that were the mainstay of family studies, researchers now looked for ways of identifying statistical associations between genomic markers and the occurrence of particular diseases, not just within families but among larger groups of people. Association studies were well established in epidemiology, where they were used to identify associations between environmental factors and increased risk of developing certain diseases, for instance. However, adapting these methods to study the genetics of common disorders was not straightforward. In order to identify a statistical association between a disease and a particular genetic marker, that marker would need to be very tightly linked to the gene that actually predisposed to that disease. Even with the growing numbers of RFLP and microsatellite markers that were available by the early 1990s, researchers realized, those markers remained too sparsely scattered on the human genome to serve as effective indicators of the presence of predisposing genes. If association methods were to have any hope of identifying genetic risk factors for complex disorders, it would first be necessary to develop human genetic linkage maps to a level of detail and resolution that far exceeded what was possible using RFLP and microsatellite markers (Bodmer, 1986; Lander and Botstein, 1986).

Consequently, for the time being, researchers sought instead to develop hybrid methods that in effect combined elements of family studies with statistical methods for identifying associations. One such method, developed in the later 1980s, involved studying large numbers of pairs of siblings affected by particular conditions in order to identify statistical associations with genetic markers that they possessed in common (Bodmer, 1986; Kruglyak and Lander, 1995; Risch, 1989, 1990a, 1990b). This method proved effective in mapping gene variants associated with a number of common diseases, including demonstrating linkage between type 1 diabetes and a region of chromosome 6 associated with the body's immune response (Davies et al., 1994).

Another method, developed around the same time, involved studying population isolates where the high degree of in-breeding and interrelatedness meant that existing linkage maps were sufficiently fine-grained to detect disease associations (Lander and Botstein, 1986: 57–59; Lander and Schork, 1994). In the event, this method proved more successful in mapping a number of rare single-gene disorders (albeit without the need to reconstruct family pedigrees) than the common complex disorders that were increasingly preoccupying medical geneticists (Houwen et al., 1994; Puffenberger et al., 1994).

By the mid-1990s further rapid developments in the field of molecular biotechnology appeared to offer a way to develop more conventional forms of association studies. New DNA sequencing technologies connected with the Human Genome Project provided increasingly rapid means of identifying much larger numbers of genomic markers than had previously been possible. By mapping single nucleotide polymorphisms (SNPs) rather than RFLPs and microsatellite variants, much higher-resolution linkage maps now became a realistic prospect. This promised a step change in the rate at which researchers could identify and map human disease genes. Indeed, for a number of the most prominent scientific advocates of the Human Genome Project this was precisely the purpose of the whole enterprise (Fortun, 1999, 2008: 35–37).

Accordingly, as groups of researchers in Europe and North America began systematically collecting, cataloguing and mapping human SNPs they came increasingly to regard association methods as the most promising means of identifying and mapping gene variants implicated in common complex disorders (Collins, Guyer and Chakravarti, 1997; Lander, 1996; Risch and Merikangas, 1996). This commitment to creating the resources necessary to undertake genetic association studies would have profound consequences for how molecular and medical geneticists thought about human genetic diversity and, ultimately, about human populations.

Capturing human genetic variation

Initially the work of identifying and cataloguing SNPs proceeded in a relatively uncoordinated fashion, with the establishment of local databases in a number of leading North American and European research centres. However, this work progressed against a backdrop of concern that researchers' access to large bodies of accumulated genomic data was threatened by moves to bring those data into private ownership. In the summer of 1997 it became apparent that a number of pharmaceutical companies were seeking to gain proprietary control of some of the leading collections of SNPs. In July of that year Abbot Laboratories announced a deal with Genset – a private company closely associated with the CEPH in Paris – to create two sets of SNPs, one for their own private research use and the other to market to other drug companies. At the same time Eric Lander, the founding director of the Massachusetts Institute of Technology's Whitehead Institute and one of the leading advocates of genetic association studies, was negotiating a deal with Bristol-Myers Squibb to create a similarly proprietary collection of SNPs to market for use in gene discovery (Marshall, 1997a).

Faced with this threat of privatization, which they feared would impede both publicly funded and commercial research into the genetics of disease and ill health, Francis Collins and other leading figures in the Human Genome Project were able to negotiate the creation in 1999 of a public-private partnership called the SNP Consortium, which included a number of leading pharmaceutical companies as well as the National Human Genome Research Institute (NHGRI) in the US and the Wellcome Trust in the UK (NHGRI, 2000). The SNP Consortium provided the organization and infrastructure to collate SNP discovery projects already under way, including a database called dbSNP which would serve as a public repository for the data generated.

More than simply collating existing SNP discovery projects, the creation of the SNP Consortium also provided an opportunity to impose a degree of order and shared purpose on those projects. In particular, it enabled the Consortium leadership to channel research in ways that were intended to promote the development of SNP maps that would be optimally configured for use in genetic association studies. This led them to seek genomic data of a quite specific kind. SNPs are points of genetic variation between individuals. In order to facilitate the discovery of SNPs, Consortium members were keen to maximise the amount of variation present in the samples they analysed. They were helped in that aim by an initiative already under way at the NHGRI. As early as 1998 the NHGRI had announced the launch of a new research with the specific purpose of facilitating the identification of SNPs. The DNA Polymorphism Discovery Resource, as it was called, comprised a collection of DNA samples from '450 U.S. residents with ancestry from all the major regions of the world' (Collins, Brooks and Chakravarti, 1998; Marshall, 1997b). With the launch of the SNP consortium in July 2000, the NHGRI provided twenty-four samples from the DNA Polymorphism Discovery Resource, taken from donors 'with diverse geographic origins', to help with its work (NHGRI, 2000). This donation proved invaluable in facilitating the search for SNPs. Initially the Consortium had aimed to generate a map of 300,000 evenly spaced SNPs within three years. In the event, by the end of 2001 it had succeeded in compiling a map detailing over one million SNPs (International SNP Map Working Group, 2001).

The NHGRI's decision to collect and study genetic data from individuals 'with diverse geographic origins' bears careful analysis. The architects of the DNA Polymorphism Discovery Resource were at pains to declare that it was not intended to support research into the biology of racial or ethnic difference; indeed, it was deliberately designed in a way that rendered it useless for such research. 'No medical, phenotypic, or ethnicity information is included' with the samples, they stressed. 'The DNA Polymorphism Discovery Resource was designed to be used to discover variants in human DNA, not to assess the frequency of variants in particular groups. Thus, the DNA Polymorphism Discovery Resource is not useful for population-specific medical or anthropological studies' (Collins, Brooks and Chakravarti, 1998: 1229–1230).

The reasons for this were partly political. American genome researchers were acutely aware that any attempt to undertake genetic research that might be seen to impinge on matters of ethnic identity would be met with suspicion. A decade earlier, building on post-war surveys of human genetic variation as well as the availability of new molecular techniques to identify gene variants, population geneticists and physical anthropologists had joined forces to launch the Human Genome Diversity Project. The aim was to sample indigenous populations around the world, particularly what geneticists regarded as endangered population isolates, in order to garner data on human origins and evolution (Reardon, 2005). The project had foundered amid charges of colonialism and racism. The architects of the DNA Polymorphism Discovery Resource therefore sought to distance themselves from that earlier debacle. They did so both by removing all racial, ethnic or geographical identifiers from the samples they collected and by presenting their work as an instance of how researchers were responding to complaints about Eurocentrism in biomedical research by deliberately including other ethnic groups (Bliss, 2012: 49–51).

The removal of ethnic and other identifiers from the DNA Polymorphism Discovery Resource was not merely a political gesture, however. It was also consistent with the purpose which the Resource was designed to serve – namely, to identify SNPs. For that purpose, there was no need to know anything about the ethnic or geographical origins of the genomes under study; it was sufficient merely to compare them and to identify the differences between them. In that respect, the Resource marked a significant break with earlier approaches to human genetic diversity. Previous anthropologically informed studies of genetic diversity, culminating in the Human Genome Diversity Project, had focused on identifying and characterizing the genetic differences between what they took to be different populations living or originating in different parts of the world – differences that were most starkly exemplified in so-called population isolates. In such studies the search for 'diversity' meant documenting how the human species had become subdivided into a number of more or less distinct evolutionary branches or backwaters. The DNA Polymorphism Discovery Resource certainly drew on such assumptions when deciding to recruit individuals whose ancestry was seen to lie in different parts of the world. But the aim in doing so was markedly different from that of earlier studies. The Resource did not seek to identify or describe genetic differences between the ancestral populations from which those individuals were supposedly drawn. On the contrary, it sought simply to maximise the number and range of genetic variants available for mapping. Beyond seeking to recruit as diverse a range of individuals as possible, the origins and ancestry of the individuals sampled were irrelevant to the aims of these studies

– hence the decision to remove geographical identifiers from the collected data. For the purposes of the DNA Polymorphism Discovery Resource, the genetic diversity of the population of the US was a useful resource, but it was not a matter for analysis.

Reconstituting populations

If the DNA Polymorphism Discovery Resource marked a step away from earlier efforts to use genetics to differentiate human populations, subsequent research initiatives decisively reasserted the old direction of travel. Following the success of the SNP Consortium in cataloguing and mapping unexpectedly large numbers of SNPs, scientists at the NHGRI proposed an even more ambitious project to identify the kinds of genomic variants that would help them to identify genes associated with common diseases. In autumn 2002 the US National Institutes of Health announced the launch of the International HapMap Project (NIH News Advisory, 2002). The aims and methods of the HapMap Project differed significantly from those adopted by the DNA Polymorphism Discovery Resource.

For one thing, where the SNP Consortium focused solely on sampling American citizens, the HapMap Project looked abroad to sample 'several populations from different ancestral geographic locations': initially Han Chinese living in Beijing, Japanese living in Tokyo, Yoruba from Ibadan in Nigeria and selected members of the Mormon families originally collected in 1980 for the CEPH project and classified within the HapMap Project as from Northern and Western Europe (International HapMap Consortium, 2003: 791). The reasoning behind this decision was again in part political. In the wake of the announcement of the first draft of the human genome in February 2001 and the growing public prestige that now attached to genome research, many feared that confining the research to the US would be seen as exclusionary. At the same time, by sampling large, culturally dominant groups in African and Asian countries it would be possible to avoid the charges of racism and colonialism that had attended the Human Genome Diversity Project. While neither of these strategies entirely avoided controversy and contestation, they were sufficient to secure participation by members of the four communities listed in the press release (Reardon, 2017: 70–93).

For another thing, the kind of genetic variation that the HapMap project sought to document differed in important ways from anything that had gone before. By the time that planning for the HapMap Project got under way, research using increasingly detailed SNP maps was revealing new details about how the human genome is structured. Among other things, it showed that DNA is organized not just into chromosomes but, at a finer level of organization, into haplotypes (Daly et al., 2001; Gabriel et al., 2002). A haplotype is a specific combination of SNPs that are not only situated close together on the genome but also tend to be inherited together across many generations – they exhibit particularly close genetic linkage, in other words. For molecular geneticists interested in mapping SNPs, and ultimately in identifying genetic variants associated with common diseases, the existence of haplotypes provided a welcome methodological shortcut: if researchers identified the presence of one or more SNPs peculiar to a particular haplotype, then they could infer with a high degree of probability what other SNPs markers were likely to be located in the immediate vicinity. Consequently, the HapMap project was organized with the express purpose of collecting not just SNPs but haplotypes as the preferred markers of human genetic variation.

However, the turn to haplotypes also opened the door to other kinds of genetic analysis. Since haplotypes are groups of genetic markers that tend to be inherited together, geneticists were able to read them not just as units of genetic variation but as indicators of common descent: if individuals share a haplotype, they must also have a common ancestor. In the context of the sampling strategy adopted by the HapMap Project this aspect of haplotypes quickly acquired a set of meanings that went well beyond the Project's professed claim to be concerned solely with variation. HapMap researchers did not just collect DNA samples from individuals; they sampled what they saw as specific populations, defined by ethnic identity and geographical location. As a result, the particular patterns of haplotypes identified in each of those populations were strongly associated from the start with particular ethnic groups and their supposedly disparate ancestral origins. As a number of commentators have observed, the particular choice of populations to study, in Africa, Asia and white North America, effectively served to reinscribe long-standing ideas about race into the findings of the HapMap Project, including the idea that different racial types could be mapped onto particular continental locations (e.g. Duster, 2015; Hamilton, 2008). More generally, the very act of assembling different groups of people to sample, then characterising the differences between those groups in terms of distinctive hereditary patterns of haplotypes, served in effect to constitute the very populations which those haplotypes were supposed to represent (Reardon, 2017: 80–82).

This concern with sampling disparate populations, and the idea that those populations were genetically different from one another in important ways, in turn resonated with another, rather different understanding of populations that was becoming increasingly salient in debates about the feasibility of association studies as a means of identifying disease genes. As we have seen, earlier family linkage methods for identifying disease genes had not involved any explicit conceptualization of populations, since such studies focused on families as the object and means of investigation. However, once geneticists began considering the possibility of conducting association studies, the language of 'populations', and particular technical ideas about those populations, became central to their work.

For at least three decades before medical geneticists began to consider adopting association methods to elucidate genetic factors in disease, epidemiologists had been refining those methods for use in identifying environmental and other causes of ill health. Central to their methodological armamentarium were so-called case-control studies. In order to identify possible causes of illness, epidemiological researchers typically compare a group of affected cases with a group of non-affected controls and seek to identify statistical associations between the occurrence of the disease and specific environmental or other factors. In the course of developing such methods epidemiologists quickly realized that false positive results can occur if the cases and controls are not sufficiently similar to one another in relevant respects. Systematic differences between cases and controls, for instance in potentially confounding factors such as age or socio-economic status, could lead to misleading statistical associations between disease and environmental or other circumstances. For this reason, as early as the 1950s epidemiologists developed tools and methodologies designed to ensure as far as possible that cases and controls embodied the same 'population structure'.

In such studies epidemiologists use the language of populations pragmatically, to refer simply to the groups of cases and controls involved in the study. 'Population' in this sense implies nothing about the background of those who take part in a study, while 'population structure' is a consequence of the way that cases and controls are selected. That usage, and its connotations, changed markedly as medical geneticists began to adopt case-control methods, and epidemiological ideas about populations ran up against ideas drawn from population genetics. Problems of confounding due to unrecognized differences between cases and controls quickly became apparent as attempts to find associations between disease and specific genetic markers began to gain momentum. For instance, a 1980s study conducted among the Pima people of Arizona initially appeared to show an association between type 2 diabetes and a particular genetic marker. However, on further analysis the association was instead judged to be 'an artifact of population admixture'. Pima people had been selected for study because they experience a much higher incidence of diabetes than white North Americans – a fact that researchers hoped would facilitate their search for predisposing genes. However, on re-examining their findings the researchers found that the non-affected controls recruited into the study reported having more white Americans among their forebears than did the affected cases, who mostly claimed to have solely Pima ancestors. The researchers concluded that 'the association was apparently because tribe members have different degrees of Caucasian ancestry'; they had been misled by their failure to select 'a control group that is perfectly matched for ethnic ancestry' (Lander and Schork, 1994: 2041–2042).

It is worth pausing to reflect on the language adopted here. It reveals an important slippage: from thinking about populations and population structure in the instrumental language of epidemiology – referring simply to those individuals who together make up a study population – to thinking about populations in terms of population genetics – referring to the larger groups of people *from which* those individuals are judged to have been drawn. It also reveals a tendency for geneticists to think about 'population structure' not simply as an artefact of the selection of cases and controls but as something that already exists in the world from which the cases and controls are selected. This is particularly clear in the way that 'population structure' was equated with 'population admixture' in the Pima diabetes study. The very notion of 'population admixture' presumed not only that the Pima people from whom the research participants were drawn represented an uneven mix of two previously distinct genetic populations – the original Pima and 'Caucasians' – but also that the cases and controls had in effect been drawn from different sub-populations with 'different degrees of Caucasian ancestry'. In genetic case-control studies, in other words, the 'populations' which non-genetic epidemiologists would in principle have understood to have been constituted through the act of selecting cases and controls now came, in practice, to be seen as representing genetic populations that existed independently of the study methodology.

Such thinking persisted as high-density SNP maps and, subsequently, haplotype maps became available and researchers began conducting much more high-powered association studies using much larger populations of cases and controls. In such large-scale studies the potentially confounding effects of population structure (in the narrow epidemiological sense) would present a constant risk of spurious association. Consequently, researchers began developing increasingly powerful statistical techniques for analysing the distribution of SNPs within study populations, in order to discern any systematic differences between cases and controls. Their arguments were marked by constant slippage between instrumental talk of study populations and realist talk of populations of origin, and between population structure and population admixture (e.g. Devlin and Roeder, 1999; Marchini, Cardon, Phillips and Donnelly, 2004; Pritchard and Donnelly, 2001). This slippage was reinforced by the rolling-out of the HapMap Project and the growing use of haplotypes to identify population structure in association studies of disease-linked genetic markers.

Since the early 2000s association studies have proliferated and expanded, attracting large-scale research funding to study genetic factors in an increasingly wide range of medical and other conditions. Analysis of haplotypes is now routinely used in such studies as a means of controlling for population structure and ensuring that cases and controls are properly matched. In principle, this need not involve making inferences about what external populations might be represented in a study. It is possible, for instance, to use haplotype analysis to ensure simply that cases are compared with haplotypically similar controls within the study population. In practice, however, haplotype analysis commonly draws on assumptions about the ancestry of study participants, and about the genetic make-up of geographically and ethnically defined populations from around the globe. The method of admixture mapping, for instance, relies on researchers not only identifying different genetic sub-populations within the study population but also attributing common ancestry and geographical origins to those sub-populations (Fujimura, Rajagopalan, Ossorio and Doksum, 2010; Fullwiley, 2008). By contrast, attributions of ancestry are not a necessary step in large-scale genome-wide association studies, which use specialized software to conduct purely statistical analyses of population structure. Even here, however, the haplotypes used to conduct such analyses typically derive from initiatives such as the HapMap Project, and hence ultimately refer back to assumptions about the differences between geographically and ethnically defined populations; while researchers often make their own assumptions about what ancestral populations they might expect to be represented in their study sample when deciding how to interpret and classify the sub-populations identified by their software. As a result, ideas of race, ethnicity and the genetic differences between populations are constantly being reinscribed in research into the genetic determinants of common disorders (Fujimura and Rajagopalan 2011; Gannett, 2014).

Conclusion

During the 1980s and 1990s efforts to identify and map genetic variants of possible significance for disease aetiology focused primarily on families. More recently, such research has shifted to include large-scale association studies in populations rather than in families. This has in turn led to the development of new methods to determine and control for population structure, which, in the case of genomic research, has come to mean the presence of sub-populations of different biological ancestry. Researchers are accordingly anxious to know about the genomic constitution not just of those populations that are the principle focus of their research but of other populations that might in effect intrude into their study samples. The implications of this have been twofold.

First, it has entailed a shift in medical thinking about human populations. Not only has it fostered a new reification of the idea of a population as something that is defined by common biological descent; it has also led to a renewed interest in finding molecular techniques for differentiating between such populations. As Joan Fujimura and Ramya Rajagopalan put it, 'contrary to emphasizing the notion that humans are all related', studies of population structure in the context of genomic association studies are 'buttressed by a logic of difference' (Fujimura and Rajagopalan, 2011, 21). This logic of difference provides a vehicle by which old and supposedly discredited biological notions of race find their way back into human genetics.

Second, this new thinking about genetic populations, and the desire to differentiate between them, has led to the rolling-out of genetic sampling on an increasingly global scale. In order to know what genes might be involved in the incidence of heart disease among the inhabitants of America or Britain, researchers now need to know about the genetic constitution of populations from Mexico to Kenya to Japan. Local studies must routinely take into account the global distribution of genes and genotypes. In this respect, research into the genetic causes of disease, wherever it is conducted, is increasingly global in its purview, even when it is local and parochial in its concerns. This has prompted a proliferation of studies, from the International HapMap Project to the Human Heredity and Health in Africa (H3Africa) Initiative (launched in 2010), designed to reveal in ever more detail the genetic make-up of populations around the world.

Advocates of such initiatives declare that they are expected to benefit the populations being studied. But, insofar as the data they produce are used in the search for disease-causing gene variants, the vast majority of that work has been oriented towards elucidating and ultimately relieving the health problems of people – especially white people – living in North America and Europe (Need and Goldstein, 2009; Popejoy and Fullerton, 2016). By comparison, the flow of medical knowledge, and of such health interventions as result from these studies, back to the world's poorer regions has been tiny. For one thing, the extent to which knowledge about genetic causes of disease among Europeans and North Americans is applicable to people with different genetic constitutions is often unclear. For another, impoverished patients and health systems simply do not have the resources to enable them to make use of the often expensive and complex interventions that modern biomedicine affords. The outcome of human genetic variation research in Africa, Asia and South America has been overwhelmingly to facilitate the development of health-related investigations and interventions among white Europeans and Americans. To the extent that this is the case, the globalization of genomic research has tended simply to reproduce the extractive relationships of neo-colonialism by extracting biological resources from the global South and realizing the value of those resources predominantly in the global North.

Acknowledgements

The research for this chapter was funded by a Wellcome Trust Senior Investigator Award in Medical Humanities WT100597MA: Making Genomic Medicine. I am grateful to research fellows Cate Heeney, Farah Huzair and Koichi Mikami for formative conversations and additional material. The chapter has benefited immeasurably from audience feedback at the conference 'From International to Global: Knowledge, Diseases and the Postwar Government of Health', Paris, 12–14 February 2015, and from discussion by the Twentieth Century Histories of Knowledge About Human Variation reading group during my time as a visiting scholar at the Max Planck Institute for the History of Science, Berlin, 21 September–18 October 2015: my thanks to Jenny Bangham, Sarah Blacker, Helen Curry, Judith Kaplan, Lara Keuck, Erika Milam and Skúli Siggurdson. Thanks especially to Jenny Reardon, Harry Campbell and Cate Heeney for their careful reading and insightful comments on earlier drafts. All remaining errors, misinterpretations, omissions and infelicities are entirely my own.

References

Bangham, Jenny (2014) 'Blood Groups and Human Groups: Collecting and Calibrating Genetic Data after World War Two', *Studies in History and Philosophy of Science Part C: Studies in History and Philosophy of Biological and Biomedical Sciences* 47 (A), 74–86.

Bangham, Jenny (2015) 'What is Race? UNESCO, Mass Communication and Human Genetics in the Early 1950s', *History of the Human Sciences* 28 (5), 80–107.

Bliss, Catherine (2012) *Race Decoded: The Genomic Fight for Social Justice.* Stanford, CA: Stanford University Press.

Bodmer, Walter F. (1986) 'Human Genetics: The Molecular Challenge', *Cold Spring Harbor Symposia on Quantitative Biology* 51, 1–13.

Botstein, David, Raymond L. White, Mark Skolnick and Ronald W. Davis (1980) 'Construction of a Genetic Linkage Map in Man Using Restriction Fragment Length Polymorphisms', *American Journal of Human Genetics* 32, 314–331.

Cantor, David (2006) 'The Frustrations of Families: Henry Lynch, Heredity, and Cancer Control, 1962–1975', *Medical History* 50 (3), 279–302.

de Chadarevian, Soraya (2014) 'Chromosome Surveys of Human Populations: Between Epidemiology and Anthropology', *Studies in History and Philosophy of Science, Part C: Studies in History and Philosophy of Biological and Biomedical Sciences* 47 (A), 87–96.

Collins, Francis S., Lisa D. Brooks and Aravinda Chakravarti (1998) 'A DNA Polymorphism Discovery Resource for Research on Human Genetic Variation', *Genome Research* 8, 1229–1231.

Collins, Francis S., Mark S. Guyer and Aravinda Chakravarti (1997) 'Variations on a Theme: Cataloguing Human DNA Sequence Variation', *Science* 278 (5343), 1580–1581

Comfort, Nathaniel (2012) *The Science of Human Perfection: How Genes Became the Heart of American Medicine*. New Haven, CT: Yale University Press.

Daly, Mark J. et al. (2001) 'High-Resolution Haplotype Structure in the Human Genome', *Nature Genetics* 29, 229–232.

Dausset, Jean et al. (1990) 'Centre d'Etude Du Polymorphisme Humain (CEPH): Collaborative Genetic Mapping of the Human Genome', *Genomics* 6 (3), 575–577.

Davies, June L. et al. (1994) 'A Genome-Wide Search for Human Type 1 Diabetes Susceptibility Genes', *Nature* 371, 130–136.

Devlin, Bernard J. and Kathryn Roeder (1999) 'Genomic Control for Association Studies', *Biometrics* 55, 997–1004.

Donis-Keller, Helen et al. (1987) 'A Genetic Linkage Map of the Human Genome', *Cell* 51, 319–337.

Duster, Troy (2015) 'A Post-Genomic Surprise: The Molecular Reinscription of Race in Science, Law and Medicine', *British Journal of Sociology* 66 (1), 1–27.

Fortun, Mike (1999) 'Projecting Speed Genomics', in *The Practices of Human Genetics: International and Interdisciplinary Perspectives*, ed. Mike Fortun and Everett Mendelsohn (pp. 25–48). Dordrecht: Kluwer.

Fortun, Mike (2008) *Promising Genomics: Iceland and DeCODE Genetics in a World of Speculation*. Berkeley; Los Angeles; London: University of California Press.

Fujimura, Joan H., Ramya Rajagopalan, Pilar N. Ossorio and Kjell A. Doksum (2010) 'Race and Ancestry: Operationalizing Populations in Human Genetic Variation Studies', in *What's the Use of Race? Modern*

Governance and the Biology of Difference, ed. Ian Whitmarsh and David S. Jones (pp. 169–186). Cambridge, MA: MIT Press.

Fujimura, Joan H. and Ramya Rajagopalan (2011) 'Different Differences: The Use of 'Genetic Ancestry' Versus Race in Biomedical Human Genetic Research', *Social Studies of Science* 41 (1), 5–30.

Fullwiley, Duana (2008) 'The Biologistical Construction of Race: 'Admixture' Technology and the New Genetic Medicine', *Social Studies of Science* 38 (5), 695–735.

Gabriel, Stacey B. et al. (2002) 'The structure of haplotype blocks in the human genome', *Science* 296, 2225–2229.

Gannett, Lisa (2001) 'Racism and Human Genome Diversity Research: The Ethical Limits of "Population Thinking"', *Philosophy of Science* 68 (3), Supplement: Proceedings of the 2000 Biennial Meeting of the Philosophy of Science Association: S479–S492.

Gannett, Lisa (2003) 'Making Populations: Bounding Genes in Space and Time', *Philosophy of Science* 70 (5), 989–1001.

Gannett, Lisa (2014) 'Biogeographical Ancestry and Race', *Studies in History and Philosophy of Science Part C: Studies in History and Philosophy of Biological and Biomedical Sciences* 47 (A), 173–184.

Gannett, Lisa and James A. Griesemer (2004) 'The ABO Blood Groups: Mapping the History and Geography of Genes in *Homo Sapiens*', in *Classical Genetic Research and Its Legacy: The Mapping Cultures of Twentieth-Century Genetics*, ed. Hans-Jörg Rheinberger and Jean-Paul Gaudillière (pp. 119–172). Abingdon: Routledge.

Gaudillière, Jean-Paul (2000) 'Mendelism and Medicine: Controlling Human Inheritance in Local Contexts, 1920–1960', *Comptes Rendus de l'Académie Des Sciences. Série III: Sciences de la Vie* 323, 1117–1126.

Gormley, Melinda (2009) 'Scientific Discrimination and the Activist Scientist: L. C. Dunn and the Professionalization of Genetics and Human Genetics in the United States', *Journal of the History of Biology* 42, 33–72.

Gurdasani, Deepti et al. (2015) 'The African Genome Variation Project Shapes Medical Genetics in Africa', *Nature* 517 (7534), 327–332.

Gusella, James F. et al. (1983) 'A Polymorphic DNA Marker Genetically Linked to Huntington's Disease', *Nature* 306 (5940), 234–238.

Hamilton, Jennifer A. (2008) 'Revitalizing Difference in the HapMap: Race and Contemporary Human Genetic Variation Research', *Journal of Law and Medical Ethic* 36 (3), 371–477.

Harper, Peter S. (2008) *A Short History of Medical Genetics*. Oxford: Oxford University Press.

Houwen, R. H. J. et al. (1994) 'Genome Scanning by Searching for Shared Segments: Mapping a Gene for Benign Recurrent Intrahepatic Cholestasis', *Nature Genetics* 8, 380–386.

International HapMap Consortium (2003) 'The International HapMap Project', *Nature* 426, 789–796.
International SNP Map Working Group (2001) 'A Map of Human Genome Sequence Variation Containing 1.42 Million Single Nucleotide Polymorphisms', *Nature* 409, 928–933.
Jones, Emma M. and E. M. Tansey (eds) (2015) *Human Gene Mapping Workshops c.1973–c.1991*. Wellcome Witnesses to Contemporary Medicine, vol. 54. London: Queen Mary University of London.
Kan, Yuet Wai and Andreé M. Dozy (1978) 'Polymorphism of DNA Sequence Adjacent to Human β-Globin Structural Gene: Relationship to Sickle Mutation', *Proceedings of the National Academy of Sciences* 75, 5631–5635.
Kaufmann, Alain (2004) 'Mapping the Human Genome at Généthon Laboratory: The French Muscular Dystrophy Association and the Politics of the Gene', in *From Molecular Genetics to Genomics: The Mapping Cultures of Twentieth-Century Genetics*, ed. Jean-Paul Gaudillière and Hans-Jörg Rheinberger (pp. 129–157). Abingdon and New York: Routledge.
Knowlton, Robert G. et al. (1985) 'A Polymorphic DNA Marker Linked to Cystic Fibrosis is Located on Chromosome 7', *Nature* 318, 380–382.
Kohler, Robert E. (1994) *Lords of the Fly: Drosophila Genetics and the Experimental Life*. Chicago: University of Chicago Press.
Kruglyak, Leonid (2008) 'The Road to Genome-Wide Association Studies', *Nature Reviews Genetics* 9 (4), 314–318.
Kruglyak, Leonid and Eric S. Lander (1995) 'Complete Multipoint Sib-Pair Analysis of Qualitative and Quantitative Traits', *American Journal of Human Genetics* 57, 439–454.
Lander, Eric S. (1996) 'The New Genomics: Global Views of Biology', *Science* 274, 536–539.
Lander, Eric S. and David Botstein (1986) 'Mapping Complex Genetic Traits in Humans: New Methods Using a Complete RFLP Linkage Map', *Cold Spring Harbor Symposia on Quantitative Biology* 51, 49–62.
Lander, Eric S. and N. J. Schork (1994) 'Genetic Dissection of Complex Traits', *Science* 265 (5181), 2037–2048.
Lindee, M. Susan (2003) 'Voices of the Dead: James Neel's Amerindian Studies', in *Lost Paradises and the Ethics of Research and Publication*, ed. Francisco Salzano and Magedelene Hurtado (pp. 40–73). New York: Oxford University Press.
Lindee, M. Susan (2005) *Moments of Truth in Genetic Medicine*. Baltimore, MD: Johns Hopkins University Press.
Lipphardt, Veronika (2012) 'Isolates and Crosses in Human Population Genetics; or, a Contextualization of German Race Science', *Current Anthropology* 53 (Supplement 5), S69–S82.

Lipphardt, Veronika (2014) '"Geographical Distribution Patterns of Various Genes": Genetic Studies of Human Variation After 1945', *Studies in History and Philosophy of Science Part C: Studies in History and Philosophy of Biological and Biomedical Sciences* 47 (A), 50–61.

Marchini, Jonathan, Lon R. Cardon, Michael S. Phillips and Peter Donnelly (2004) 'The Effects of Human Population Structure on Large Genetic Association Studies', *Nature Genetics* 36 (5), 512–517.

Marks, Jonathan (2012) 'The Origins of Anthropological Genetics', *Current Anthropology* 53 (Supplement 5), S161–S172.

Marshall, Eliot (1997a) 'Snipping Away at Genome Patenting', *Science* 277 (5333), 1752–1753.

Marshall, Eliot (1997b) '"Playing Chicken" Over Gene Markers', *Science* 278 (5346), 2046–2048.

Necochea, Raul (2007) 'From Cancer Families to HNPCC: Henry Lynch and the Transformations of Hereditary Cancer, 1975–1999', *Bulletin of the History of Medicine* 81 (1), 267–285.

Need, Anna C. and David B. Goldstein (2009) 'Next Generation Disparities in Human Genomics: Concerns and Remedies', *Trends in Genetics* 25, 489–494.

NHGRI (2000) 'Human Genome Project and SNP Consortium Announce Collaboration to Identify New Genetic Markers for Disease', July, www.genome.gov/10001456 (accessed 10 January 2015).

NIH News Advisory (2002) 'International Consortium Launches Genetic Variation Mapping Project', October, www.genome.gov/10005336 (accessed 10 January 2015).

Nukaga, Yoshio (2002) 'Between Tradition and Innovation in New Genetics: The Continuity of Medical Pedigrees and the Development of Combination Work in the Case of Huntington's Disease', *New Genetics and Society* 21 (1), 39–64.

Popejoy, Alice B. and Stephanie M. Fullerton (2016) 'Genomics is Failing on Diversity', *Nature* 538 (7624), 161–164.

Pritchard, Jonathan K. and Peter Donnelly (2001) 'Case-Control Studies of Association in Structured or Admixed Populations', *Theoretical Population Biology* 60, 227–237.

Puffenberger, Erik G. et al. (1994) 'Identity-by-Descent and Association Mapping of a Recessive Gene for Hirschsprung Disease on Human Chromosome 13q22', *Human Molecular Genetics* 3, 1217–1225.

Rabinow, Paul (1999) *French DNA: Trouble in Paradise*. Chicago: University of Chicago Press.

Radin, Joanna (2014) 'Unfolding Epidemiological Stories: How the WHO Made Frozen Blood into a Flexible Resource for the Future', *Studies in*

History and Philosophy of Science Part C: Studies in History and Philosophy of Biological and Biomedical Sciences 47 (A), 62–73.

Reardon, Jenny (2004) 'Decoding Race and Human Difference in a Genomic Age', *Differences: A Journal of Feminist Cultural Studies* 15 (3), 38–65.

Reardon, Jenny (2005) *Race to the Finish: Identity and Governance in an Age of Genomics*. Princeton; Oxford: Princeton University Press.

Reardon, Jenny (2017) *The Postgenomic Condition: Ethics, Justice, and Knowledge After the Genome*. Chicago and London: Chicago University Press.

Rheinberger, Hans-Jörg and Jean-Paul Gaudillière (eds) (2004) *Classical Genetic Research and Its Legacy: The Mapping Cultures of Twentieth-Century Genetics*. London: Routledge.

Risch, Neil (1989) 'Genetics of IDDM: Evidence for Complex Inheritance with HLA', *Genetic Epidemiology* 6, 143–148.

Risch, Neil (1990a) 'Linkage Strategies for Genetically Complex Traits. II. The Power of Affected Relative Pairs', *American Journal of Human Genetics* 46, 229–241.

Risch, Neil (1990b) 'Linkage Strategies for Genetically Complex Traits. III. The Effect of Marker Polymorphism on Analysis of Affected Relative Pairs', *American Journal of Human Genetics* 36, 242–253.

Risch, Neil and Kathleen R. Merikangas (1996) 'The Future of Genetic Studies of Complex Human Diseases', *Science* 273, 1516–1517.

Smocovitis, Vassiliki Betty (2012) 'Humanizing Evolution: Anthropology, the Evolutionary Synthesis, and the Prehistory of Biological Anthropology, 1927–1962', *Current Anthropology* 53 (Supplement 5), S108–S125.

Solomon, Ellen and Walter F. Bodmer (1979) 'Evolution of Sickle Variant Gene', *Lancet* 313, 923.

Tsui, Lap-Chee et al. (1985) 'Cystic Fibrosis Locus Defined by a Genetically Linked Polymorphic DNA Marker', *Science* 230 (4729), 1054–1057.

Wailoo, Keith and Stephen Pemberton (2008) *The Troubled Dream of Genetic Medicine: Ethnicity and Innovation in Tay-Sachs, Cystic Fibrosis, and Sickle Cell Disease*. Baltimore: Johns Hopkins University Press.

Weissenbach, Jean et al. (1992) 'A Second-Generation Linkage Map of the Human Genome', *Nature* 359 (6398), 794–801.

Widmer, Alexandra (2014) 'Making Blood "Melanesian": Fieldwork and Isolating Techniques in Genetic Epidemiology (1963–1976)', *Studies in History and Philosophy of Science Part C: Studies in History and Philosophy of Biological and Biomedical Sciences* 47 (A), 118–129.

8

Rare genetic disease, global health and genomics: the case of R337h in Brazil

Sahra Gibbon

Introduction

The emerging relationship between genomics and a terrain of global health aligns arenas of social practice, cultural meaning and political value that might until recently have seemed antithetical. Developments in genomic research and medicine since the turn of the twenty-first century have long been associated with the promises of so-called personalized medicine, linked mostly to costly, high-end technological interventions focused on facilitating the choice of individual patients and their families who have resources or means to access and act upon genetic information (Tutton, 2014). These are health care scenarios which until recently were mostly thought to be available only in North America and Europe. Global health, by comparison, most commonly refers to populations and references a wider set of challenges to health, particularly in resource-poor contexts. Advocated solutions typically often include non-medical or non-technological interventions to address and ameliorate structural health inequalities and disparities (Beaglehole and Bonita, 2010).

The increasingly visible meeting points between genomics and global health challenge an assumed opposition between these domains, raising questions about the dynamics of their realignment and their potentially newly constituting features. These shifts reflect an emerging focus on populations and public health in the context of genomics and interlinkages between epidemiology, molecular biology, environment and human biological variation that are now being explored across a wide variety of national and transnational scientific and medical research contexts. Since the early 2000s newer and faster-sequencing 'high throughput' techniques and technologies have informed and propelled novel arenas of genetic and epigenetic research in relation to a dynamic field of enquiry that is focused on a diverse range of disease conditions, directly tying genomics to large-scale global epidemiological studies. This approach is increasingly seen as central to addressing infectious disease and the growing economic and social burden of common chronic diseases such as cancer, diabetes and cardiovascular disease in developed and emerging economies, where the focus is very much on the generation and multi-utility of large-scale databases (see, for instance, Mayer-Schonberger and Cukier, 2013).

Examining the ways that genomic health care and research are being newly configured as a pathway to global health remains a central task for social scientists (Gibbon, Kilshaw and Sleeboom-Faulkner, 2018) in examining how it is both 'a product of and vector for globalization' (Beaudevin and Pordié, 2015). Contributing to an emerging arena of enquiry, this chapter first outlines the context in which a focus on rare genetic disease – which has long been a central feature of genetic medicine – is now being reinvigorated in relation to global health. I show how efforts to address what has been described as a 'genomic health divide' and 'missing heritability' inform and justify moves to examine and extend genetic research among so-called 'underserved' populations. At the same time these efforts are underpinned by 'new regimes of innovation' (Callon, 2007) and the pursuit of niche markets facilitated by moves towards disease stratification. It is against this backdrop that an interest in rare genetic disease has become a central 'platform' (Keating and Cambrosio, 2003) for the translation of genomics. Drawing on Rabeharisoa et al.'s (2014) discussion of how a contrasting 'politics of numbers and singularisation' has come to define the varieties of activism constituted by rare-disease patient organizations, I examine how this provides a particular point of leverage for examining the intersection between rare genetic disease and global health agendas. I explore the local articulation of these dynamics by examining the 'biomedical collectives' (Cambrosio et al., 2014) that have mobilized around a particular biomarker identified at high population frequency in Brazil and associated with a normally 'rare' cancer syndrome. In examining how rareness and the variety of politics it enfolds is defined and put to work across terrains of local and global social action, this chapter shows how it is a constituting feature of the partial and sometimes uneasy alignments between genomics and global health.

Inequities, genomics and global health

Questions of inequalities and genomics were explicitly articulated in the broad context of the WHO's Human Genetics Programme in the early and mid-2000s. While the importance of genetics to health has been recognized by the WHO since the 1960s, the more recent focus on genomics has centred on widening access to and use of research resources and medical genetic services in efforts to address what has been described as a 'genomic divide between rich and poor' (see, for instance, Thorsteinsdottir et al., 2003). Calls to 'bridge global inequities' are articulated in terms of the need for economic investment, research, clinical provision and the global expansion of genomic services and technologies.

Recent work in anthropology has also examined how the issue of genomics and health inequalities has become part of the landscape in which an expanding scope for genetic research and medicine is currently unfolding. This has brought to light the complex intersections between health disparities, genomics and racial justice, particularly in the US (Bliss, 2012; Lee, 2013). Nonetheless, how a discourse of social justice becomes articulated in relation to genomics is dependent on particular social and often colonial and post-colonial histories of 'race', racism, multiculturalism, public health provision and the changing governance of research vis-à-vis health disparities, as well as transnational collaborations (Fullwiley, 2011; Fullwiley and Gibbon, 2018; Santos et al., 2014; Wade et al., 2014; Whitmarsh, 2008).

A concern with inequalities, social justice and genomics has more recently become explicitly aligned around a notion of 'missing heritability'. While often defined as the currently 'unknown' genetic variants and epigenetic pathways that may be associated with a range of increasingly common diseases (Maher, 2008), this is a concept which has also been deployed in calls to widen programmes of genetic research to global health care arenas outside Western Europe and North America. This was a key message of an article published in 2011 in *Nature Genetics* entitled 'Genomics for the World', where calls for genotype information from 'minority populations' and 'other ethnic groups' were emphasized to ensure that 'those most in need are not the last to receive the benefits of genetic research' (Bustamante et al., 2011). An emphasis on the 'humanitarian' dimensions of expanding genomic research to include 'underserved groups' brings to the fore how questions of social justice and inclusion are central to situating genomics as a pathway to global health, while also raising challenges and concerns about the ethical complexities of the 'research/care hybrids' that emerge at this interface (Gibbon and Prainsack, 2018; see also Gibbon and Aureliano, 2018).[1] At the same time, as Steve Sturdy points out (chapter 7, this volume), efforts to diversify and widen the parameters of participation in genomic research beyond North America and Europe are also about ensuring the relevance and accuracy of genomic data for populations in those same regions. From this perspective, 'missing heritability' encompasses not only currently unknown genetic variation or the urgency of genotyping diverse populations for 'humanitarian' reasons in terms of widening access to participation and resources, but also the ongoing viability of genomic science and medicine for 'Western' consumer markets.

Stratified medicine and regimes of innovation

The way that an expanding terrain of genomics and global health brings to the fore questions of social justice and inequalities in considering as yet 'unknown' genetic variants relevant to particular populations or geographical regions also reflects the increasing moves towards disease stratification. Described sometimes as 'precision medicine', or more ubiquitously as 'personalised medicine' (Tutton, 2014), this is an emerging but still mainly promissory dimension of genomic health care. It has nevertheless been made most visible in the field of oncology, at the 'tangled intersection' (Keating and Cambrosio, 2013) between translational research and clinical care. It is a meeting point which entails transformations not only in the expanded 'biomedical collectives' (Bourret, 2005) that now coalesce around the field of cancer genetics but also in cancer patienthood, described by Kerr and Cunningham-Burley (2015) as 'embodied innovation'.[2] While the stated aim of stratified medicine is to move beyond a 'one size fits all' approach to more accurately characterize patient populations and subgroups for better and improved targeted treatment, this is also tied to what Callon (2007) has described as 'new regimes of innovation' and the development of differentiated 'niche' pharmaceutical markets. In a global context this means taking account of how the necessary involvement and needs of different populations are positioned as vital components in fulfilling (and making equitable) the future health promises of genomic knowledge. It entails, as Rayna Rapp points out, examining how 'different publics are becoming part of exquisitely stratified research populations that now serve as potential global resources and market beneficiaries' (Rapp, 2013: 574).

In an arena where the global and globalizing vectors and terrains of genomic research and medicine are unfolding, a focus on 'rare' genetic disease is being explicitly situated as central to the translation of genomic health care and, as a result, entwined with issues of disease stratification, the development of niche markets, missing heritability and social justice.

Rare genetic disease and translating genomics

An interest in rare disease in genetic medicine is not new. With 80% of so-called rare diseases thought to be genetic in origin and many related to single gene alterations, the feasibility of a focus on rare diseases in genetics has long been recognized. What is notable is the shift in scale and scope of national and transnational initiatives addressing 'rare' disease and the way they are explicitly situated as a 'platform' for the wider application of genomics to public health, particularly in the context of large-scale, high-profile genetic research initiatives. As one scientific commentator reflecting on the application of next-generation sequencing for rare disease put it, 'hardly a day goes by where there is not another discovery of a gene for a rare disease' (Danielsson et al., 2014).

The expanded scope for newborn genetic screening in the US and the UK, which is now targeted at identifying a wider range of rare but potentially disabling conditions before symptoms develop, is extending the space of the clinic in genomic medicine (Timmermans and Buchbinder, 2012). The UK's high-profile 100,000 Genomes Project set up by Genomics England, a company established by the Department of

Health in 2012, aimed at sequencing the genomes of 100,000 people to produce a 'lasting legacy for patients, the NHS and the UK economy', has an explicit focus on so-called 'rare' diseases, as well as cancer and infectious diseases. As one of the briefing documents from Genomics England states:

> Rare diseases present an ideal opportunity to establish a platform for the application of high-throughput genomics in routine NHS practice. As a group rare diseases affect 6% of the UK population and more than 85% are caused by a single gene defect. Many are chronic and associated with substantial morbidity and premature mortality. Early diagnosis enables accurate genetic counselling and prevention and may lead to new treatments based on genetic stratification. (Genomics England Science Working Group, 2015)

Nevertheless, definitions of rare disease vary. In the US rareness is defined in terms of prevalence, a condition that affects less than 200,000 people. While the European Commission's definition relies on a prevalence threshold which is lower (1 in 2,000), but further qualified with reference to conditions that are 'life-threatening or chronically debilitating'. Taking this variability into account, WHO figures suggest that there are 6,000–7,000 rare diseases worldwide and that they affect 8% of the world's population. As a number of social scientists working in this arena have illuminated, the estimated numbers of those affected play a key role not only in framing scientific and medical interest and gaining resources for research but also in the way that publics and patients engage with rare genetic disease.

'The politics of numbers and singularisation': rare genetic diseases and activist communities

Work examining the role of patient organizations has been of particular importance in examining the changing meaning and significance of 'rare' disease. Exploring and comparing patient organizations, mainly in Europe and the US, a number of social scientists have tracked how 'rareness' is variably produced and engaged with by different patient organizations and activist communities in efforts to raise awareness, access resources and, in some cases, shape research trajectories (Rabeharisoa, 2003; Rabeharisoa and Callon, 2004; Rabeharisoa et al., 2014;

Huyard, 2009). Much of this work describes how certain of these groups, particularly during the 1990s, participated in making equivalent the notion of rare disease and patients' exclusion, so that rareness appeared as the cause of discrimination against patients and, as a result, became a political issue. As the work of Huyard also demonstrates, such activities led in the US to a lowering of the threshold for clinical trials involving so-called orphan drugs and diseases, and thereby succeeded in transforming 'uncommon disorders' into 'rare diseases' (Huyard, 2009). Rabeharisoa et al. suggest that efforts on the part of patients to make visible the 'undone science' of rare disease, based on principles of fairness, equity and social justice, have until recently very much relied on 'politics of numbers' (Rabeharisoa et al., 2014). One of the messages consistently articulated by many patient groups is that while individual 'rare' diseases may indeed be rare, the total numbers affected in this way are significant and have a detrimental impact on public health. This is a discourse that is strongly reflected not only in the publicity material of patient organizations but also, more recently, in the UK government's Strategy for Rare Diseases, which states:

> The total number of rare diseases is steadily increasing because genetic research is beginning to explain disease patterns that we did not understand before. Research shows that 1 in 17 people will suffer from a rare disease at some point. In the UK this means more than 3 million people will have a rare disease – so rare diseases are not that rare. They represent a significant cause of illness, making considerable demand on the resources and capacity of the NHS and other care services. (UK Department of Health, 2013: 5)

Nevertheless, activism around the quantification and aggregation of rare diseases stands in contrast to a different strategy adopted by other patient organizations, characterized by what Rabeharisoa et al. (2014) describe as a 'politics of singularisation'. Here a clear-cut stable definition of rareness is substituted for an attention to specificity as part of an ongoing 'qualification of relevant differences and similarities', such that patients and the collectives they belong to are 'simultaneously constituted and continuously reassembled' (Rabeharisoa et al., 2014: 212). They suggest that this is not necessarily about individualization or reductionist biologization of rare disease but instead can potentially lead to the exact opposite. That is, different specificities in the biological pathways, signs, symptoms and experience of rare disease conditions can result in the formation of new collectives or new pathways to access broader and diverse research terrains beyond the parameters of any specific rare disease.[3] At the same time there is an acknowledgement by these authors that 'singularisation' of rare genetic disease can serve to strengthen and is also itself nurtured by the opening up of niche pharmaceutical markets.

This research is very much focused on the role of patient organizations and their relationship to scientific expertise in reconstituting the meaning and significance of 'rareness'. Nevertheless, I would suggest that a discussion of the politics of 'numbers' and 'singularisation', provides a point of leverage in examining how an expanding interest in rare genetic disease in the context of globalizing genomic medicine is being calibrated to local and global contexts in specific ways. To further illuminate these dynamics I turn to the case of rare genetic disease in Brazil, drawing on ethnographic research undertaken in the domain of cancer genetics in the south of the country.[4]

Oncogenética in Brazil

The development of specialist cancer genetics clinics and services in Brazil has emerged since the mid-2000s, in the wealthier and relatively more economically developed southern part of the country. With extremely high rates of breast and prostate cancer in these regions (equivalent to the population prevalence in the US map; INCA, 2014), it is a location which not only reflects regional differences in cancer incidence but also relative differences in wealth and, to some extent, access to health care services. The scope of Brazilian clinical cancer genetics, while increasingly fuelled by the growth of private genetic testing and screening, is also very much centrally linked to university hospitals and specialist research units. Nevertheless, it is limited by the lack of integration of genetic services more generally into the public health system, and consequently constituted by a degree of dependency on research collaborations. As a result there is a close and dynamic relationship between emerging clinical services, which are focused on promoting a neglected preventative approach to health care through risk-based interventions, and research objectives linked to national and transnational collaborations (Aureliano, 2015; Gibbon, 2015b). The undefined boundary between cancer genetic research and clinical services has been noted as a significant feature of cancer genetics elsewhere (Hallowell et al., 2009; Kerr and Cunningham-Burley, 2015), and is more widely indicative of the 'clinical collectives' that have become a defining feature of translational research in cancer genetics (Bourret et al., 2005; Cambrosio et al., 2014). Nevertheless, the relative lack of integration of cancer genetics into public health services and a dependence on research funding (both national and transnational) make such boundaries more than usually fluid and, as a result, complex in resource-poor contexts such as Brazil.

One of the articulations around the necessity for cancer genetics in Brazil has been an emphasis on identifying what are described as the currently 'unknown' parameters of cancer genetic risk in Brazil and the need to *padronizar*, or standardize, testing protocols and criteria in order to know the genetic variants that pose a risk for the Brazilian population. This emphasis in part reflects the questions of social justice, 'underserved populations' and 'missing heritability' that are characteristic of a global genomic health agenda outlined above. This lacuna has also fuelled research efforts to identify common so-called 'founder mutations' that might be of relevance to certain populations or that might explain the higher incidence of cancer in specific regions of the country. The economic logic that lies behind these goals, related to reduced costs, was an aspect that the health professionals I met constantly emphasized in their work.

Nevertheless, efforts to identify the currently unknown genetic parameters also reflect the real everyday challenges of making meaningful sense of genetic risk in the clinic, given the potentially limited applicability of risk estimates and protocols derived from elsewhere. This challenge was reflected in the guidelines for managing familial cancer in Brazil produced by the Instituto Nacional de Cancer (INCA), which stated;

> The Brazilian population has its own characteristics due to its ethnic and cultural diversity, with regional variations, which makes impossible the application of data obtained in other regions of the world about the risks and frequency of mutations related to hereditary cancer syndromes. This highlights the need to know and characterise these mutations and optimise clinical screening in ways that consider the particular aspects of our population. (INCA, 2009)

On numerous occasions I witnessed the extensive efforts of clinicians who, having obtained a family history from the patient in the clinic, would painstakingly work their way through various online risk-modelling tools. They would flick hesitantly between the models and risk-calculating programmes available through international online portals, seeing if there were significant differences depending on the criteria entered, trying to decide which risk estimate best fitted their patient and to make decisions on recommended interventions and care protocols. One of the stumbling blocks was often what to put in the box related to ancestry, particularly when they often felt that the narrow categories of 'Caucasian' or 'African American' or 'Ashkenazi Jewish' (often the only 'ethnic' identifiers that were available to them in the risk-modelling tools) simply didn't fit the profile of the patients they encountered in the clinics. In the context of high-profile genetic research fields such as those focused on the two BRCA genes associated with an increased risk of breast cancer, the concern to *padronizar* Brazilian cancer genetics has informed an ambivalent engagement with, and also a critique of, the relevance and meaning of categories of population difference.[5]

In Brazilian cancer genetics, therefore, clinical need is constituted with reference to an 'underserved population' in the context of mostly yet 'to-be-discovered' genetic components or the uncertainty of variants with unknown significance that may ultimately contribute to understanding and addressing the high and growing incidence of cancer in Brazil as part of a neglected preventative approach to health (Gibbon, 2015b).

The case of R337h

In the expanding field of *oncogenética* in Brazil there has been a growing interest in a particular genetic variant known as R337h and located on the TP53 gene, which has been described very explicitly in scientific literature and clinical discourse as a 'Brazilian Founder Mutation'. Germ-line mutations on the TP53 are infrequent – estimated to be around 1 in 5,000 in the US – but have been linked to a rare cancer syndrome known as Li-Fraumeni, whose carriers are estimated to have a 90% lifetime chance of developing a range of cancers (Malkin et al., 1990).

In the early 2000s a series of Brazilian studies began to suggest that a specific germ-line mutation on the TP53 gene, R337h, was particularly common in the south of the country, with research associating this mutation with ostensibly rare cancers specifically in children, as well a range of more common adult cancers such as breast cancer.

The variant R337h was initially associated with a high incidence of adrenocortical cancers in children in the southern state of Parana (Ribeiro et al., 2001). Since 2007 Brazilian researchers have also linked the mutation to breast and other types of cancer in the neighbouring southern states of Rio Grande do Sul and Sao Paulo (Achatz Waddington et al., 2007). While generating a good deal of controversy and debate in genetic research communities in Brazil, the state of Parana's decision in 2006 to screen all newborn children through the '*teste do pezinho*', or blood spot test, for R337h has also revealed the high population prevalence of the mutation, found in 1 in 300 of all children screened, or 0.3% of the population. This finding has been replicated elsewhere by much smaller studies investigating the high incidence of breast cancer in southern Brazil (Achatz et al., 2009; Giacomazzi et al., 2014).

The purported population prevalence of R337h in the south of Brazil has had a key part in efforts by members of the Brazilian cancer genetic community to constitute it as a significant public health problem, where a 'politics of numbers' has been used to generate national and international interest in and engagement with this area of scientific research. The purported global rareness of adrenocortical cancers in children and of Li-Fraumeni syndrome has been constantly juxtaposed against the estimate that 1 in 300 people in particular regions of Brazil are carriers of the genetic variant, thereby providing foundation to the claim that these normally 'rare' cancers and cancer syndromes are not so rare in Brazil. In one national meeting which brought together leading researchers working in the field of Brazilian cancer genetics in 2011, R337h was discussed in terms of its being likely to account for between 2,000 and 4,000 cases of cancer a year and was described in terms of having 'clear implications for public health'. Accounts in popular national newspapers have similarly emphasized the numbers of those likely to be carrying R337h in the south of Brazil, as compared to the limited numbers of persons affected elsewhere – quoted in one article as the '280 persons affected by the syndrome in the world' (Tarantino, 2011). In the clinical contexts that I observed there was a similar emphasis on the numbers likely affected. While the question of 'rareness' globally was emphasized less than the frequency of R337h in the southern part of Brazil, there was nonetheless a certain ambiguity in the way that the specific known regional frequency of the mutation was conveyed in clinical contexts. For example, R337h was often described to patients as the 'Brazilian mutation' (*mutação brasileira*) that was common 'among us' (*comun em nosso meia*).[6]

The dynamic movement between both a relational association and *difference* with the 'rare' Li-Fraumeni syndrome by Brazilian researchers has therefore been central to underlining the relevance of R337h. It is also notable how the identification of the variant R337h in Brazil has also been used by Li-Fraumeni researchers and patient organizations in the US as evidence of the growing incidence of the syndrome or to highlight the neglected needs of those with the condition, as well as to help to constitute the syndrome as a platform for broader-terrain scientific research. This was reflected in the comments about R337h research in Brazil by the researcher who first described the syndrome, Joseph Fraumeni. In an article in a popular Brazilian journal reflecting on the relevance of R337h he stated: 'we are rethinking the study of rare diseases with this syndrome ... it's a way of advancing our study of the molecular causes of cancer' (cited in Tarantino, 2011).

Nevertheless, the exact population prevalence of R337h in Brazil, its association with different cancers and the epigenetic or environmental factors associated with its variable expression are all subject to ongoing research and debate. Here the reconfiguration of 'rareness' is variably contested within different sectors of cancer research and paediatrics in Brazil. The shift to describe R337h in Brazil as a 'conditional cancer pre-disposing mutation' (Giacomazzi et al., 2014) whose expression is dependent on as yet unknown environmental components reflects a terrain in which the association with cancer risk continues even as new epidemiological findings about the prevalence and penetrance of R337h make estimations of that risk more rather than less complex. Moreover, while some researchers in São Paulo and Porto Alegre have emphasized data which shows an association with breast cancer, arguing that testing for R337h must be included in programmes of hereditary breast and ovarian cancer screening in the southern regions, researchers in Parana continue to contest these findings, suggesting a lack of evidence for an association of the variant with Li-Fraumeni syndrome and maintaining that R337h is associated primarily with adrenocortical cancer in children. This has been met with openly published critiques by those who see the newborn population screening for this mutation in the state of Parana as irresponsible, given the association which they claim to have identified between R337h and the Li-Fraumeni cancer syndrome, in which carriers can develop a range of cancers as both children and adults (see Achatz et al., 2009).

These scenarios are characteristic of what Rabeharisoa and Bourret (2009) have described in terms of the 'clinic of mutations' that increasingly characterise genomic medicine where bioclinical entities, similar to R337h, are subject to often contested and temporary qualifications. At the same time these debates and controversies haven't obstructed attempts at innovation in ways that reveal the niche marketing possibilities that are nascent in these developments. This includes the initial efforts of one São Paulo university to develop cheap rapid-testing technology for mass population screening of R337h (see Arruda and Sensato, 2013). While the development of this technology was linked to patent approval stated for use in public hospitals, the development of such techniques would likely also be extremely viable in the commercial sector in Brazil.

Below I provide a further illustration of these dynamics and the way that a 'politics of numbers and singularisation' were put to work and made evident during one key event in my fieldwork where the regional frequency of R337h, as well as its variable expression and metabolic pathways, were used for particular kinds of mobilizations at the dynamic interface between patients and researchers.

Mobilizing patients and research

In June 2011 I participated in a unique event in the southern city of Porto Alegre, where a number of the families of those who had been identified as carrying the particular mutation R337h were invited to what was described as a 'family meeting' set up by the researchers in the public hospital. About forty or so patients were waiting in the auditorium when I arrived, sitting mostly in small groups, with one large extended family – a number of whom had travelled overnight by bus from the interior parts of the state, paid for by the hospital. In the presentations that took up most of the morning information was provided about the discovery of the mutation, its frequency in the south of the country and its association with what was previously thought to be a 'rare' cancer syndrome, Li-Fraumeni. Some qualification was provided to patients that the syndrome in Brazil appeared to be different from the classic syndrome identified elsewhere, with suggestions that this particular germ-line mutation did not necessarily confer the high 90% lifetime risk of developing cancers associated with TP53 germ-line mutations in Europe and the US. A large map of the region identifying the clusters where those carrying the mutation had been identified was shown. The researcher in fact pointed out how all identified carriers had, as she put it, 'a common ancestor' because of the association of the syndrome with a founder mutation and given its seemingly high regional population presence. While the map was of interest to many of the patients and families their questions were much more focused on what was being done to treat and prevent the disease, to provide care and resources for those in the areas that were most affected. Was there, as one person asked, going to be a vaccine? The response of clinicians was hesitant but centred on how this research was about developing preventative health care strategies for affected communities. Another patient, talking about his gratitude for the research that was taking place in relation to the families, said 'you are doing so much for us, what can we do for you?'[7]

The final part of the morning was a talk from a younger scientist who was carrying out new research looking at the function of R337h. He explained its importance in helping to know why, as he put it, the 'risk was different for carriers of the mutation in Brazil' and 'why some people had the mutation but never developed cancer'. He explained how he was investigating the possibility that R337h could be specifically associated in Brazil with metabolism and diet and that this might mean that they would be able to develop a therapy, even a dietary supplement, to treat those identified as carriers. The meeting then finished, and those who wanted to participate in this new avenue of research were invited to come and donate blood and sign the consent form, and all were invited to a lunch provided by the hospital.

In these exchanges we see the extent to which not only the activism of researchers is engaged in co-producing patient communities but also the different ways in which 'rareness' is assembled such that R337h is simultaneously *connected to* and *differentiated from* the syndrome known as Li-Fraumeni. We see how an emphasis on the specificity of the condition in Brazil becomes a means of enlisting local research subjects while also engaging a wider international research community. The possibility presented to the patients that the particular expression of R337h in Brazil might be linked to metabolic function (discussed in terms of diet with the patients and families) was of great interest to the families and also a new and exciting research avenue for the scientific team. My discussions with different members of the team later revealed how a great deal of hope was pinned on explaining the wide variability in the expression of the disease in Brazil, particularly given that many of those identified as carrying the mutation had not been diagnosed with cancers. At the same time this novel research trajectory also places the focus on what is globally an ostensibly rare condition within a broader paradigm of transnational cancer research centred on examining the genetic and epigenetic pathways that link metabolism and cancer more generally. It was significant that this was a research trajectory which had already involved collaborations with research teams in the US.

But other mobilizations were also visible in the exchanges that took place at this event, which came to light in a conversation I had with one of the participants whom I met in the weeks following this meeting.

Jose is part of a large extended family that had had multiple cases of cancer and many deaths. He had been at the meeting with several members of his extended family, a number of whom had been identified as carrying the R337h mutation although he himself had not had cancer and was a not a carrier of R337h. When we met he talked specifically about how this had been an opportunity to exchange experiences, and also to concretise a sense of group identity.[8] This was how Jose talked about his experiences:

> When I saw everyone entering we saw that they were all persons who had the mutation. We all looked at each other ... But we slowly got used to each other. We saw that we are not alone with this. I said to my family 'let's talk with them, exchange our ideas'. That lunch together was a real opportunity to chat and get to know each other. So it was really good. Someone from the group who has the same fault can find a way through this, or reassure others. Really, this group, we have something in common. It's a really strong connection. It's genetic whether you like it or not, not family but a genetic connection. So I think we have to try and get together using the internet so we can talk about these things.

The case of R337h in Brazil is illuminating for thinking about how the focus on rare genetic diseases as part of a globalizing terrain of expanding genomic medicine is also subject to a process of localization. Here 'rareness' is being dynamically formulated at the interface with questions of social justice linked to underserved communities at the same time that it is conjoined to research exploring the viability of 'rare genetic disease' to account for and sustain research into 'missing heritability'. The aggregation and disaggregation of similarities and differences with the Li-Fraumeni syndrome that is unfolding around R337h, far from destabilizing, in fact becomes a vector through which specificity can be highlighted and used to mobilise research and potentially, as the account outlined above suggests, also nurture nascent patient activism. In this sense the case of R337h in Brazil illuminates the local and global processes by which 'rare' genetic diseases are becoming a 'platform' through which new 'clinical collectives' are being constituted. This not only aligns and extends national and transnational research communities but also reconfigures the role of patients and research participants.

Conclusion

This chapter has examined the complex vectors around which a resurgent interest in 'rare' genetic disease is being formulated across a diverse terrain of research, forging new if still partial realignments between genomics and global health where questions of social justice intersect with disease stratification, but also with the potential for market innovation. In this context work to address 'undone' science and bridge the 'genomic health divide' becomes entangled with efforts to assemble 'rare genetic disease' as a platform for genomic and increasingly postgenomic research in the hope-filled pursuit of translational research, personal medicine and preventative health.

Drawing on one particular case study, the case of R337h in Brazil and the Li-Fraumeni syndrome, I have shown how a 'politics of numbers and singularisation' provide a point of leverage in examining how a global focus on rare genetic disease is unfolding in specific locations. Crucially, the activist communities at stake in these developments include clinicians and researchers pursuing both transnational research *and* the rights of 'underserved' communities as they attempt to stabilise risk associated with mostly 'unknown' genetic variants. At the same time patients or families seeking rights to care, treatment and intervention are not passive actors but are recruited and enrolled into research, although this is often in an effort to secure hard-to-access basic medical services and care. In conclusion I provide further reflection on other developments in Brazil that are also transforming and reconstituting the meaning of 'rare' genetic diseases where specific kinds of patient activism and citizenship are implicated.

In November 2013 a popular television network that broadcasts from the Brazilian Senate dedicated a whole programme to rare genetic diseases.[9] It brought explicit attention to the high numbers of those thought to be affected by such conditions in Brazil, between 13 million and 15 million people according to the Ministry of Health. More significantly, presenting in detail the experience of a few families with these conditions, focus was drawn to the lack of appropriate attention on rare diseases in public and private health care. The stories of a family with hereditary ataxia and a young teenage girl with cystic fibrosis were outlined, highlighting not only the dearth of appropriate health care available to them but also how, in each case, the families had pursued or were pursuing judicial cases in the courts to ensure that they had the resources, medication and facilities to care for their loved ones. As Waleska Aureliano suggests in her analysis, the message conveyed by the programme is that the recent upsurge of judicialization in Brazil is linked to limited and inadequate medical resources for rare and, in many cases, genetic disease (Aureliano, 2015).

The rapid growth of health judicialization in Brazil has been noted by a number of commentators (Aureliano and Gibbon, 2020; Biehl, 2013; Diniz, 2009), illuminating a phenomenon in which thousands of Brazilian patients across different social and economic classes are now effectively suing the government for the right to health care resources. This includes not only medication but also other treatments, examinations and tests, predicated on a constitutional commitment in Brazil to provide health care for all. It is significant that the first such successful cases of judicialization have occurred in the context of participation in clinical trial research for medication related to mainly rare genetic conditions, although patients are pursuing, and very often successfully obtaining, the right to health care resources for a wide range of conditions. In 2013 a geneticist in cancer genetics clinics in the south of the country commented that of the thirty or so patients they see each week in the public health hospital at least one is going through a judicialization process to secure rights, mostly, in these cases, for genetic testing – procedures which are not currently available via the public health system.

While the role of the pharmaceutical industry in promoting judicial cases for access to drugs and treatment points to the complex ways in which judicialization has been and is developing in Brazil (Diniz, 2009), we must also, as Aureliano highlights, be careful not to assume that this 'judicialised citizenship' is necessarily predicated on the individual's 'rights' to manage one's health (Aureliano, 2015). She suggests, rather, that judicialization might more often be seen as a struggle for better health care from the state, supported in this case by a responsive judicial system (see also Grudzinski, 2013). In this sense these are developments that point to the relevance of 'bio-legitimacy' (Fassin, 2009) as a central feature of how citizenship and activism are situated in relation to the politics of rare genetic disease in Brazil (see also Guilherme Do Valle and Gibbon, 2015).

It is at the same time hard to see the recent upsurge in cases of judicialization as separate from the 2014 Brazilian federal directive to form a national policy for the Comprehensive Care of People with Rare Disease, especially as this followed intensive lobbying by scientists and patient associations (Aureliano, 2015; Melo et al., 2015). While the consequences of this new directive are still unfolding, it marks a watershed in the attention to rare genetic disease within the Brazilian public health system, ensuring, in theory, comprehensive diagnosis and clinical attention for up to ten rare genetic diseases in reference centres located across the country. Those identified as carriers of R337h associated with Li-Fraumeni syndrome in Brazil are currently not included. However, just as patient litigants in Brazil have been seeking rights to genetic testing for the BRCA genes it will be important to monitor how the new directive for rare genetic diseases unfolds and whether we will see the emergence of judicial demand either for genetic testing in the case of R337h or for carriers, in order to obtain routine screening as part of preventative health care approach.[10] It highlights the need for ongoing and critical examination of who and what gets excluded and included in the shifting scientific and medical focus on rare genetic disease, as the local and global dynamics of genomic research and health care become ever more complexly entwined.

Notes

1 See Lakoff (2010) for further discussion of how the expansion of 'humanitarian biomedicine' has brought the specific issue of 'neglected disease' to public prominence.
2 See also Bourret et al., 2014.
3 One illustrative exampled discussed in the paper by Rabeharisoa et al. includes a patient association in France concerned with extremely rare autoimmune disease linked to bone marrow depression. The organization PNH chose not to align itself with larger rare disease umbrella organizations but instead to emphasize the uniqueness of the condition. This enabled them to develop strong connections with a particular specialist hospital who were subsequently contacted by an American pharma company to test a new class of immunosuppressants which the patient association supported, ensuring that the drug was brought to market in the shortest time possible (Rabeharisoa et al., 2014: 207).
4 This included ethnographic research working with and alongside patients, practitioners and scientists in mostly public cancer genetics clinics in three major cities in the southern part of the country during research that was mainly undertaken from 2010 to 2012. My principal focus in this research has been on examining the interface between international agendas for cancer genetics research and questions of population difference and genetic ancestry, the historical and contemporary politics of public health in Brazil and the variable understandings of genomics and embodied risk for cancer among patients and their families.
5 My research in Brazil suggests that these population categories are made relevant through diverse registers of meaning. On the one hand, the regional specificity of the migratory histories of the southern part of the country is made evident. Yet this research is also explained in relation to, and itself becomes evidence of, the ubiquity of population mixture in Brazil, popularly but unevenly associated with a discourse of Brazilian nationhood and identity (Mozersky and Gibbon, 2014). Elsewhere I have argued, along with others (see, for instance, Wade et al., 2014), that this movement and mobility in the way that particular categories of population difference are simultaneously incorporated but also reconfigured and sometimes rejected in Brazilian cancer genetics must be understood in terms of the constantly 'situated meaning and utility' (Shim et al., 2014: 18) of genetic ancestry (see, for instance, Gibbon, 2015a).

6 See Gibbon (2015a) for further discussion.
7 Such comments illustrate not only the willingness of some patients to participate in and contribute to the research but the dynamics of the exchange on which medical research is often predicated in contexts where the terrain of health care is uneven and inequitable. In this way many patients without health insurance and dependent on precarious public health can, through participation in research, gain access to both real and perceived care in terms of additional screening and monitoring (Gibbon, 2015b; see also Petryna, 2009).
8 Something that may have been partly a result of the researchers' suggestion in the presentations that all who were carriers of R337h had a 'common ancestor'.
9 I am extremely grateful to Waleska Aureliano for bringing this programme to my attention.
10 This is particularly so when one of the key messages of those involved in this field of cancer genetics research in Brazil, focused on R337h, is that regular and routine monitoring and screening of carriers could reduce not only cancer mortality but also treatment costs.

References

Achatz, M., Hainaut, P., and Ashton-Prolla, P. (2009) 'Highly prevalent TP53 mutation predisposing to many cancers in the Brazilian population: a case for newborn screening?', *Lancet Oncology* 10 (9), 920–925.

Achatz Waddington, M. I., O. Magali, F. Le Calvez, G. L. Martel-Planche, A. Lopes, B. Mauro Rossi, P. Ashton-Prolla et al. (2007) 'The TP53 mutation R337h is associated with Li-Fraumeni and Li-Fraumeni like syndromes in Brazilian families', *Cancer Letters* 245, 96–102.

Arruda, A. and Sensato, V. (2013) 'Kit deteca mutacao genetica em tipos de cancer padiatrico', *Jornal da Unicamp* 567, 2.

Aureliano, W. (2015) 'Health and the value of inheritance', *Vibrant: Virtual Brazilian Anthropology* 12 (1), 109–140.

Aureliano, W. and Gibbon, S. (2020) 'Judicialisation and the politics of rare disease in Brazil: re-thinking activism and inequalities', in *Critical Medical Anthropology. Perspectives in/from Latin America*, ed. Gamlin, J., Gibbon, S., Sesia, P. and Berrio, L. (pp. 248–270). London: UCL Press.

Beaglehole, R. and Bonita, R. (2010) 'What is global health?', *Global Health Action* 3 (10), 5142–5143.

Beaudevin, C. and Pordié, L. (2015) 'Diversion and globalisation in biomedical technologies', special issue of *Medical Anthropology: Cross Cultural Studies in Health and Illness* 35 (1), 1–4.

Biehl, J. (2013) 'The judicialization of biopolitics: claming the right to pharmaceuticals in Brazilian courts', *American Ethnologist* 40 (3), 419–436.
Bliss, C. (2012) *Race Decoded: The Genomic Fight for Social Justice*. Stanford: Stanford University Press.
Bourret, P. (2005) 'BRCA patients and clinical collectives. New configurations of action in cancer genetics practices', *Social Studies of Science* 35 (1), 41–68.
Bustamante, C. D., De La Vega, M. and Burchard, E. G. (2011) 'Genomics for the world', *Nature* 475 (7355), 163–165.
Callon, M. (2007) 'An essay on the growing contribution of economic markets to the proliferation of the social', *Theory, Culture & Society* 24 (7–8), 139–163.
Cambrosio, A. et al. (2014) 'Big data and the collective turn in biomedicine. How should we analyze post-genomic practices?' *Tecnhoscienza Italian Journal of Science and Technology Studies* 5 (1), 11–43.
Danielsson, K. et al. (2014) 'Next generation sequencing applied to rare diseases genomic', *Expert Review of Molecular Diagnostics* 14 (4), 469–487.
Diniz, D. (2009) 'Judicialização de Medicamentos no SUS: memorial ao STF', *Série ANIS, Letras Livres* IX (66), 1–5.
Fassin, D. (2009) 'Another politics of life is possible', *Theory, Culture, and Society* 2 (65), 44–60.
Fullwiley, D. (2011) *The Encultured Gene: Sickle Cell Health Politics and Biological Difference in West Africa*. Princeton, NJ: Princeton University Press.
Fullwiley, D. and Gibbon, S. (2018) 'Genomics in emerging and developing economies', in *Handbook of Genomics Health and Society*, ed. Gibbon, S. et al. (pp. 228–239). London: Routledge.
Genomics England Science Working Group (2015) Appendix 2: Rare Diseases, www.genomicsengland.co.uk/download/science-working-group-appendix-2-rare-diseases/.
Giacomazzi, I. et al. (2014) 'Prevalence of TP53 p.R337H mutation in breast cancer patients in Brazil' *PLOS One* 9 (6), e99893.
Gibbon, S. (2015a) 'Translating population difference: the use and re-use of genetic ancestry in Brazilian cancer genetics', *Medical Anthropology* 9, 1–15.
Gibbon, S. (2015b) 'Anticipating prevention: constituting clinical need, rights and resources in Brazilian cancer genetics', in *Anthropologies of Cancer in Transnational Worlds*, ed. Mathews, H. F., Burke, N. and Kampriani, E. (pp. 68–86). New York: Routledge.
Gibbon, S. and Aureliano, W. (2018) 'Inclusion and exclusion in the globalisation of genomics; the case of rare genetic disease in Brazil', *Anthropology and Medicine* 25 (1), 11–29.

Gibbon, S. and Prainsack, B. (2018) 'Section Four: Diversity and Justice' in *Handbook of Genomics, Health and Society*, ed. Gibbon, S. et al. (pp. 179–181). London: Routledge.

Gibbon, S., Kilshaw, S. and Sleeboom-Faulkner, M. (2018) 'Genomics and genetic medicine: pathways to global health', special issue of *Anthropology and Medicine* 25 (1), 30–46.

Grudzinski, R. (2013) 'A Nossa Batalha é Fazer o Governo Trabalhar: estudo etnográfico acerca das práticas de governo de uma associação de pacientes'. Unpublished Masters dissertation, Federal University of Rio Grand do Sul.

Guilherme Do Valle, C. and Gibbon, S. (2015) 'Introduction. Health illness, biosocialities and culture', *Vibrant: Virtual Brazilian Anthropology* 12 (1), 67–74.

Hallowell, N., Cooke, S., Crawford, G., Parker, M. and Lucassen, A. (2009) 'Distinguishing research from clinical care in cancer genetics: Theoretical justifications and practical strategies', *Social Science and Medicine* 68, 2010–2017.

Huyard, C. (2009) 'How did uncommon disorders become "rare diseases"? history of a boundary object', *Sociology of Health and Illness* 31 (4), 463–477.

INCA (Instituto Nacional de Cancer) (2009) *Rede Nacional de Câncer Familial*. Rio de Janeiro: Ministerio de Saúde.

INCA (2014) *Estimativa. Incidencia de Cancer no Brasil*, www.inca.gov.br/estimativa/2014/index.asp.

Keating, P. and Cambrosio, A. (2003) *Biomedical Platforms. Realigning the Normal and the Pathological in Late TwentiethCentury Medicine*. (Cambridge, MA: MIT Press.

Keating, P. and Cambrosio, A. (2013) '21st oncology: a tangled web', *The Lancet* 392, e45–e46.

Kerr, A. and Cunningham-Burley, S. (2015) 'Embodied innovation and regulation of medical technoscience: transformations in cancer patienthood', *Law, Innovation and Technology* 7 (2), 187–205.

Lakoff, A. (2010) 'Two regimes of global health', *Humanity: An International Journal of Human Rights, Humanitarianism and Development* 1 (1), 59–79.

Lee, S. (2013) 'The political economy of personalized medicine, health disparities and race', in *Anthropology of Race: Genes, Biology and Culture*, ed. Hartigan, J. (pp. 151–169). Santa Fe, NM: School for Advanced Research Press.

Maher, B. (2008) 'Personal genomes: The case of missing heritability', *Nature* 456, 18–21.

Mayer-Schonberger, V. and Cukier, K. (2013) *Big Data: A Revolution That Will Transform How We Live, Work and Think*. London: John Murray Publisher.

Malkin, D. et al. (1990) 'Germ line p53 mutations in a familial syndrome of breast cancer, sarcomas, and other neoplasms', *Science* 250 (4985), 1233–1238.
Melo, D. G., de Paula, P.M, de Araujo Rodrigues, S., Retto da Silva de Avo, L., Maria Ramos Germano, C. and Marcos Piva Demarzo, M. (2015) 'Genetics in primary health care and the National Policy on Comprehensive Care for People with Rare Diseases in Brazil: opportunities and challenges for professional education', *Journal of Community Genetics* 6, 231–240.
Mozersky, J. and Gibbon, S. (2014) 'Mapping Jewish identities: migratory histories and the transnational re-framing of "Ashkenazi BRCA mutations" in the UK and Brazil', in *Breast Cancer Gene Research and Medical Practices: Transnational Perspectives in the Time BRCA*, ed. Gibbon, S., Joseph, G., Mozersky, J., zur Nieden, A. and Palfner, S. (pp. 35–57). London: Routledge.
Petryna, A. (2009) *When Experiments Travel: Clinical Trials and the Global Search for Human Subjects*. Princeton, NJ: Princeton University Press.
Rabeharisoa, V. (2003) 'The struggle against neuromuscular diseases in France and the emergence of the 'partnership model' of patient organisation', *Social Science and Medicine* 57 (11), 2127–2136.
Rabeharisoa, V. and Bourret, P. (2009) 'Stating and weighting evidence in biomedicine: comparing clinical practices in cancer genetics and psychiatric genetics', *Social Studies of Science* 39 (5), 691–715.
Rabeharisoa, V. and Callon, M. (2004) 'Patients and scientists in French muscular dystrophy research', in *States of Knowledge. The Co-Production of Science and Social Order*, ed. Jasanoff, S. (pp. 142–160). London and New York: Routledge.
Rabeharisoa, V., Callon, M., Marques Filipe, A., Arriscado Nunes, J., Paterson, F. and Vergnaud, F. (2014) 'From "politics of numbers" to "politics of singularisation": patients' activism and engagement in research on rare diseases in France and Portugal', *Biosocieties* 9 (2), 194–221.
Rapp, R. (2013) 'Thinking through public health genomics', *Medical Anthropology Quarterly* 27 (4), 573–576.
Ribeiro, R. et al. (2001) 'An inherited P53 mutation that contributes in a tissue specific manner to paediatric adrenocortical carcinoma', *Proceedings of the National Academy of Sciences, USA* 98 (16), 9330–9335.
Santos, R. V., Silva, G. and Gibbon, S. (2014) 'Pharmacogenomics, human genetic diversity and the incorporation and rejection of color/race', *Biosocieties* 21, 1–22.
Shim, J. K., Ackerman, S. L., Darling, K. W., Hiatt, R. A. and Lee, S. S. (2014) 'Race and ancestry in the age of inclusion: technique and meaning in postgenomics science', *Journal of Health Behaviour* 55 (4), 504–18.
Tarantino, M. (2011) 'Mais vulneráveis ao cancer', *Istoé*, 9 March, 72–77.

Thorsteinsdottir, H. et al. (2003) 'Genomic knowledge', in *Global Public Goods for Health. Health Economic and Public Health Perspectives*, ed. Smith, R. et al. Oxford: Oxford University Press.

Timmermans, S. and Buchbinder, M. (2012) *Saving Babies? The Consequences of Newborn Genetic Screening*. Chicago: University of Chicago Press.

Tutton, R. (2014) *Genomics and the Re-imagining of Personalised medicine*. Farnham: Ashgate Publishing.

UK Department of Health (2013) *UK Strategy for Rare Diseases*, https://www.gov.uk/government/publications/rare-diseases-strategy.

Wade, P., Lopez-Beltran, C., Restrepo, E. and Ventura Santos, R. (eds) (2014) *Mestizo Genomics. Race Mixture, Nation and Science in Latin America*. Durham, NC and London: Duke University Press.

Whitmarsh, I. (2008) *Biomedical Ambiguity: Race, Asthma, and the Contested Meaning of Genetic Research in the Caribbean*. Ithaca, NY: Cornell University Press.

9

The World Health Organization's response to Ebola in historical perspective

Nitsan Chorev

Introduction

The 2014–16 outbreak of Ebola in West Africa was the largest and most alarming outbreak of the disease since the virus was first discovered in 1976. The outbreak resulted in more than 28,600 cases of Ebola and 11,325 deaths, almost all of them in Guinea, Liberia and Sierra Leone.[1] It took two and a half years from the discovery of the first case to successfully fight the epidemic, in part because the initial measures that were put in place to slow its spread and treat those who were infected were inadequate. Many criticisms of the dire situation at that stage pointed to the WHO (Turshen and Tefera, 2017). This specialized agency of the UN has a leadership position on global health matters, but its initial reaction to Ebola was considered by many to be 'shamefully slow' (New York Times Editorial Board, 2014).

According to the International Health Regulations, which were most recently revised by member states of the WHO in 2005,[2] any human cases of Ebola must be reported to the WHO within twenty-four hours. Such a report should then trigger a response from the Organization. That response, however, was late to happen. The first case to be identified as Ebola was in March 2014, in Guinea. Already in April, Dr Keiji Fukuda, then the Assistant Director-General at the WHO responsible for Health Security and the Environment, stated that 'This is one of the most challenging Ebola outbreaks that we have ever faced'. But he also expressed confidence that it would be controlled.[3] It took more than three months for the WHO to convene a meeting of regional health ministers and open a regional coordination centre. In June, Médecins sans Frontières (MSF) pronounced the epidemic 'out of control',[4] but it was only in August – five months after the first case had been identified, and after almost 1,000 people had died – that the WHO Director-General, Dr Margaret Chan, formally declared Ebola a public health emergency of international concern.[5] Aid workers and health authorities on the ground complained that during those five months they saw no signs of WHO officials in charge of handling the escalating outbreak (Flynn and Nebehay, 2014).

The complaints and criticisms, especially earlier on, were somewhat over the top. And after August 2014, it is important to note, the WHO's activities were more effective. The Organization provided guidance and technical support for overall coordination, surveillance and data collection. It was also involved to some extent in the training of health workers, the provision of hospital beds and the refurbishing of clinics. In July 2015 it published a report by an Ebola Interim Assessment Panel which was intended to bring about improvements in the WHO's response to future outbreaks.[6] Still, the delayed response made it so much more difficult to effectively control the disease. It allowed the disease to spread through villages and to densely populated cities, making it almost impossible to put into practice the measures necessary to contain Ebola – namely, tracing those infected and people they have been in contact with – and much more difficult to end the outbreak.

Indeed, many WHO officials agree that they should have detected the severity of the situation earlier and 'could have responded faster'.[7] For example, the report by the Ebola Interim Assessment Panel concluded in no uncertain terms that 'The Ebola crisis [...] exposed organizational failings in the functioning of the WHO'. Director-General Chan, who was initially reluctant to take responsibility, stated in her address to the World Health Assembly in 2017 that the agency was too slow to 'recognize that the virus, during its first appearance in West Africa, would behave very differently than during past outbreaks in central Africa, where the virus was rare but familiar and containment measures were well-rehearsed'; she also stated that she was 'personally accountable'. That came later, however. WHO officials' first response to the criticism aimed at the Organization's limited range of activities in the face of the crisis was to assert that this was not the WHO's job. Francis Kasolo, head of a WHO regional Ebola response centre set up in Guinea, was reported as saying, 'We're a public health agency not a clinical management agency' (Flynn and Nebehay, 2014). And Director-General Chan insisted that the WHO's job was limited to helping governments respond better, not doing it for them (Sengupta, 2015). Even more bluntly, Dr Chan said that it was a 'fantasy' to think of the WHO as a first responder ready to lead the fight against deadly outbreaks around the world (Fink, 2014a).

Why did the WHO not respond faster? And, central to the discussion in this chapter, why did it insist on a limited role, that of guidance and coordination, even once it realized the severity of the situation? In what follows I argue that the WHO's response to the Ebola was a particularly dramatic manifestation of a transformation – in priorities, practices and rhetoric – that took place back in the 1990s. This transformation was orchestrated by the WHO bureaucracy as a strategic response to external neoliberal pressures. As a result of adapting to external impositions *strategically*, the WHO bureaucracy was able to avoid a complete neoliberal turnaround and preserve some of its interests. Maybe most importantly, the WHO was able to maintain its central concern with health at the global level. It was also able to redefine its own position in the new 'global health architecture' in a way that did not completely marginalize it. But this came at a cost. And the inability to effectively respond to the Ebola epidemic offers one manifestation of what that cost entails.

The delayed response

There is a surprising consensus on why the WHO did not respond to the spread of Ebola faster. Newspaper editorials, public health experts and amateur bloggers all seem to agree on what caused the delayed reaction. They all suggest that the WHO's budgetary constraints, combined with its shifting priorities away from communicable diseases, have resulted in the fact that its budget for outbreaks and crises has sharply declined, leading to shrinking manpower and lost capacity for adequate response (Park, 2014; Sack et al., 2014; Turshen and Tefera, 2017).

Commentators also mentioned, with some empathy, that the timing made things worse, as the Organization was overstretched by concurrent health care crises, including the MERS virus in Saudi Arabia, a new avian influenza A strain in China and polio in war-torn Syria (Sack et al., 2014). Another often-cited speculation, which rightly considers the political and not only the bureaucratic dimensions of the Organization, was that the WHO was hesitant in its response to Ebola because when swine flu broke out in 2009 and Director-General Chan declared it a pandemic she was criticized for overreacting and for pandering to pharmaceutical firms (Flynn and Nebehay, 2014).

While they were relatively understanding when it came to organizational or even political considerations, commentators were less empathetic to officials' assertions that the WHO's tasks were limited to coordination and guidance (Sengupta, 2015). Commentators were particularly critical of the concept used to justify the WHO's reliance on countries' own monitoring, that of 'ownership'.

This list of explanations – and the normative evaluations attached to them – is persuasive. There is no doubt, for example, that budgetary constraints and shifting priorities affected the WHO's response to Ebola. And there are also good reasons for critics not to be convinced by what could seem like an overly legalistic response. After all, the WHO's reputation was made largely when it went beyond coordination and technical guidance – for example, when it led ambitious global programmes, like those to eradicate smallpox or polio. In addition, relying on domestic authorities in the affected countries in the name of 'ownership' seems tragically futile. Authorities in the affected countries initially denied the situation, contributing to the international community's slow recognition of the gravity of the crisis; and lack of administrative and medical infrastructure in the affected countries was one of the main reasons to why, even once the WHO and others had identified the severity of the situation, it was so difficult to control the spread of the disease.

But the discussion so far has simply focused on the immediate and observable causes. As important, I argue, is to understand the historical conditions leading to the shift in the priorities and capabilities of the WHO, and leading to a changing perception of the WHO regarding what it is and what it is not expected to achieve. What is required, in addition, is a historical-sociological account of the conditions leading the WHO to become, at least in the case of Ebola, a failed coordinating entity.

The neoliberal turn of the 1990s

A historical-sociological account of the conditions leading to the failed response to Ebola takes us back to the 1990s – when, in response to a global 'neoliberal turn', the WHO went through a transformation that resulted in new priorities, practices and rhetoric.[8]

The neoliberal turn is most broadly understood as the embrace of economic reforms that draw on the self-efficiency of the market and minimize governmental interventions, and include trade liberalization, the privatization of public services and deep budget cuts, including in health. The turn to such neoliberal policies began with the introduction of economic reforms in Chile, the US and the UK. A similar logic was later also adopted by many other governments, independently of their political inclinations or their country's level of economic development (Harvey, 2005). Many developing countries, in particular, had little choice. In the midst of a major debt crisis, starting in the early 1980s, developing countries were offered much-needed loans from the World Bank and the International Monetary Fund (IMF), but only under the condition that they would adopt market-liberalizing reforms (Babb, 2009). According to some accounts, not only the World Bank and the IMF but also other international organizations strongly advocated neoliberal policies (Cox, 1986).

But others also convincingly insist that neoliberalism is not a hegemonic, all-encompassing order. Instead, what happens on the ground is what we can call 'actually existing neoliberalism' (Brenner and Theodore, 2002), which allows for plurality in the experience of neoliberalism – including at the international level. This plurality is in part a result, I argue, of the ability of international organizations – including the WHO – to respond strategically, and therefore selectively, to pressures to adhere to the neoliberal logic.

Indeed, international organizations are not passive transmission belts for policy prescriptions developed elsewhere; and they do have some influence on the content of policies which they adopt and help to disseminate. Also in response to neoliberal pressures, international organizations have been active participants in the construction of their own policies. Specifically, the WHO bureaucracy pushed for an agenda that, while seemingly compatible with external neoliberal pressures, was also in line with its own organizational interests and considerations.

No doubt the WHO – like any other international organization – is vulnerable to external pressures. It is the member states, rather than the WHO bureaucracy, that decide on how much funding to commit to the WHO and that vote at the World Health Assembly on WHO policies. The WHO bureaucracy is particularly sensitive to the demands of wealthy member states, and also to the positions held by the more prestigious and better-funded international organizations, including the World Bank. The conventional expectation is therefore that an international organization would comply with demands made by external actors independently of the organization's internal preferences. By complying, the organization may successfully manage its relations with the external environment – but potentially at the expense of its own internal preferences. Alternatively, international bureaucracies may refuse to adhere to external demands (Oliver, 1991). However, such resistance may undermine the organization's relations with external actors, which might penalize the organization in response.

In addition to compliance and resistance, when international bureaucracies are confronted with demands that are in conflict with their own agenda they may try to minimize the potential tension by way of 'strategic' responses. By 'strategic' I mean responses that involve an attempt to restructure or redefine the meaning of the external demands so that the response can also conform to the organization's own agenda. In cases of *strategic compliance*, the international bureaucracy adheres to the external expectations, but only after giving them a meaning that is still compatible with the external demands but that can also be reconciled with the organization's independent goals. In cases of *strategic resistance*, the international bureaucracy reframes the dominant logic so that it is no longer expected to conform to it. The international bureaucracy, in such cases, is able to rely on reframed principles to justify its refusal to comply. In this way, the organization can resist without risking retaliation.

The WHO, I argue, often utilized strategic responses instead of complying with or explicitly resisting the neoliberal turn. In the section below I describe what the WHO was able to protect through strategic adaptation. But this strategy is also not without a cost. The case of Ebola tells us about the price paid.

Strategic adaptation to neoliberal pressures

The WHO was established in 1948 as a specialized agency of the UN. It was considered to be one of the more reputable UN agencies, but its initial experience of the neoliberal turn was quite a negative one, as the adoption of neoliberal policies by external actors triggered a set of crises, threatening the WHO's authority, funds and legitimacy.

The WHO suffered *authority crisis* as the World Bank – a much better-funded and more influential organization – became interested in public health issues. The Bank advocated policies that directly competed with and – partly due to their neoliberal orientation – often contradicted the WHO's own policies. For example, the Bank recommended budget cuts in the public health sector, charging user fees for public health services and privatization of public health services. All of these policies were in sharp contrast to the position of the WHO at that time (Abbasi, 1999).

The World Bank also threatened the WHO's authority by adopting a new way for deciding on health priorities. Traditionally, the WHO was mostly interested in helping those 'most in need' – populations with the most severe health needs and the least ability to afford health care. In the 1970s and 1980s it was also concerned with affordability and called for reliance on 'appropriate technology', but this was relevant to the decision how to treat, not whom to treat. The World Bank came with a very different formula that, in a way, reversed that order. Concretely, World Bank economists formalized a way to calculate the 'return' (in 'productive life saved') for every dollar invested in health programmes and announced that priority should be given to the most cost-effective interventions (World Bank, 1993). The result was a very different set of priorities than those held dear by WHO officials.

In addition to an authority crisis, the WHO also suffered a *financial crisis*. The financial crisis was the result of a number of related developments. Most importantly, following pressures from the US and many European countries, the WHO had agreed in the early 1990s to freeze its budget, which in the past had increased by at least 10% annually. This decline in mandatory payments was partly compensated for by an increase in voluntary contributions. Between the 1970s and 1990s voluntary funds increased from 20% to almost 60% of the total budget (Lee, 2009). In 2015 voluntary contributions made up almost 80% of total WHO funds.[9] While they saved the WHO from an even worse financial fate, voluntary funds were 'earmarked' for specific programmes and in this way allowed a small number of rich countries to bypass the World Health Assembly, which deepened the subordination of the WHO to the whims of a small number of countries.

Initially, the WHO bureaucracy was unable to offer an adequate response to either the authority or the financial crises. The Organization was partly paralysed, no doubt, due to a concurrent *legitimacy crisis*. Traditionally, the WHO was considered to be a well-functioning agency, but that changed in 1988 when Dr Hiroshi Nakajima was elected Director-General with the support of developing countries and against the position of the US. The accusations made against Dr Nakajima were often personal, but concerns were also expressed regarding weak leadership and poor management. Typical titles in leading medical journals during this time included, 'What Role for WHO in the 1990s?' (Lee and Walt, 1992), 'WHO in Crisis' (Godlee, 1994a) and 'WHO in Retreat' (Godlee, 1994b).

Starting in 1998, under the new leadership of Director-General Gro Harlem Brundtland, the WHO bureaucracy tried a new response to the external pressures, which would allow it to regain the funds, authority and legitimacy it had lost. Under Dr Brundtland the WHO abandoned existing policies and embraced new ones. But it was hardly a passive recipient of neoliberal prescriptions imposed from above. Instead, the WHO bureaucracy was able to restructure neoliberal themes into policies and programmes somewhat different than what the US government or the World Bank would have supported, and in that way preserved at least some of its core organizational agenda. Three policy realms illustrate the strategic adaptation of the WHO: the repositioning of health in the international agenda; setting of WHO priorities; and a structural reorganization in response to a new health architecture.

Repositioning health (health in economic terms)
As part of the neoliberal turn foreign aid became increasingly focused on the narrow goal of economic growth, with the assumption that other policy concerns, including health, would automatically improve with

economic growth. This approach directly undermined organizations like the WHO that were responsible for issues that were now of lesser concern.

In strategically responding to this threat, the WHO abandoned its traditional assertion that health was an issue that should be addressed in its own right and accepted the focus on economic growth as the main – or even only – target. However, it also adopted the provocative premise that health was good for economic growth.

It was not easy to convince donor countries that health was good for economic growth. After all, neoliberal economists conceived of health as an 'unproductive consumer of public budgets', while Director-General Brundtland wanted to argue that wise investment in health was 'key to productivity itself' (quoted in Birmingham, 1999). For the message to be effective, the promise of growth had to be convincing. As Brundtland said in an interview: 'Anchoring health on the development agenda (...) involves not just reaching the minds of people who have decision-making power (...) but also increasing the evidence base so that you have convincing arguments' (Yamey, 2002a). To make the arguments convincing she wanted to make sure that the WHO was able 'to stress the importance of health in economic terms' (Birmingham, 1999). To provide the economic evidence needed, in January 2000 the WHO established the Commission on Macroeconomics and Health (CMH).

The CMH was chaired by the economist Jeffrey Sachs, who was formerly one of the central advocates of neoliberal reforms in Latin America and the former Soviet Union. Other members of the Commission included former ministers of finance, and officers from the World Bank, the IMF, and the World Trade Organization. Clearly, the CMH was an attempt to co-opt leading economists by giving them the task of presenting the WHO's position on the economic importance of health.

Brundtland's instructions to CMH members made her expectations explicit: 'Placing health at the heart of the development agenda. This is the purpose of the Commission.' She then elaborated: 'That poverty causes ill health is well known. But good health can fuel the engine of development [...] This is the case we have to make' (Brundtland, 2000). CMH members complied. The Commission's report provided economic evidence showing that health was one of the most effective means by which to achieve economic development. The CMH's policy recommendations were exactly what the WHO wanted to hear: the way to achieve economic growth was a massive injection of financial resources into health services (CMH, 2001).

What did the WHO achieve? By justifying investment in health with the promise for economic growth, the WHO bureaucracy capitulated to the reductionist logic of neoliberalism which saw development through the narrow lens of economic thinking. It no longer defended the notion of social development that allowed, for example, concern with individuals' quality of life independently of the economic realm. At the same time, the WHO did not simply submit to the economic reasoning of the World Bank. Instead, it restructured that very reasoning. The World Bank emphasized the causal link between poverty and disease in order to prioritize economic development. The WHO report turned the World Bank's reasoning on its head by insisting that improvement in health was necessary to achieving the goal of economic growth. Altering the meaning of the neoliberal premises before adhering to them allowed the WHO to reject the World Bank's call for budget cuts in the public health sector and to use the goal of economic growth to call, on the contrary, for greater investment in public health.

Setting priorities (cost-effectiveness)

Framing the importance of health in a language that economists would appreciate gave legitimacy to more investment in health. But investment in what? How to decide on priorities? As mentioned earlier, the World Bank prioritized health programmes based on cost-effective calculations. In response, the WHO, too, shifted its priorities to programmes that offered cost-effective interventions. The main indication of the shift from equity to cost-effectiveness at the WHO was the *World Health Report 2000*. This report rejected the WHO's previous focus on those most in need and endorsed cost-effectiveness as a tool for priority setting. An algorithm in the report offers a list of questions that should guide governments' decision-making process, and recommends interventions that benefit the poor if and only if they are cost-effective (WHO, 2000: 55).

In responding to external expectations, then, the WHO shifted its priorities so that they focused on health problems (1) that had positive impact on economic development and (2) for which cost-effective interventions were available. Such considerations gave priority to chronic diseases – which are considered easier to prevent, and which affect a growing segment of the world population – over communicable diseases. But, again, the WHO restructured the policies that it adopted. While it followed these new imperatives, the WHO's top new priorities were still three major communicable diseases often affecting those most in need, namely, malaria, tuberculosis and HIV/AIDS.[10] All three initiatives were presented as contributing to development. For example, one slogan for the malaria initiative was, 'Roll Back Malaria, Roll in Development', and the first Executive Director for the initiative, Dr David Nabarro, stated: 'Malaria is taking costly bites out of Africa ... It is feasting on the health and development of African children and it is draining the life out of African economies' (cited in Packard, 2009). In addition, for all three diseases, cost-effectiveness was used to justify the choice of preferred interventions. These interventions at times reflected a neoliberal logic. In the malaria initiative, for example, the WHO initially supported for-profit markets for selling bed-nets rather than distributing them for free. But attention was given not only to cost-effective preventive measures but also to costly treatment, including in the case of HIV/AIDS, where the WHO helped to 'neutralize' a World Trade Organization agreement on intellectual property rights and to use it in support of generic versions of patented medicines (Chorev, 2012b). In other words, while adopting a cost-effective logic the WHO was able to draw on it to justify interventions that the WHO was likely to support independently of any economic calculations.

Repositioning the WHO (coordination and ownership)
In addition to being forced to justify investment in health and to rethink health priorities, another major challenge for the WHO was the emergence of a new 'global health architecture' (Walt, Spicer and Buse, 2009). In line with the neoliberal distrust in states-led and politicized organizations, and with the neoliberal faith in market-oriented solutions and in actors with market-based experience, new types of international health entities have emerged. The Global Fund to Fight AIDS, Tuberculosis and Malaria reflected the desire of donor countries to free themselves from the political logic of UN agencies. Also popular were the so-called public-private partnerships (Richter, 2004; Walt and Buse, 2000). These were collaborations between public and private actors, often targeting one particular goal such as the development or

distribution of drugs. Notable health partnerships include Medicines for Malaria Venture (MMV), International AIDS Vaccine Initiative (IAVI), Drugs for Neglected Diseases initiative (DND*i*) and the GAVI Alliance, among many others. These partnerships were mostly funded by private foundations, did not have all governments as members and, if they welcomed the WHO at all, it was often as a non-voting member (Chorev, Andia and Ciplet, 2014).

As a result, the WHO, which used to be the only authority on international health issues, has become one actor among many. As of 2014, one report counted forty bilateral donors, twenty-five UN agencies, twenty global and regional funds and ninety global initiatives that targeted health activities. Combined, they had more than $31 billion in funding (Renwick and Johnson, 2014). The WHO's annual budget was as little as 5% of this sum.

The WHO sought different ways by which to respond to the challenge. For example, it welcomed NGOs, private foundations and private industries as more active participants in WHO deliberations. It also established its own public-private partnerships in which it could maintain a relatively central role. More importantly, however, the WHO re-emphasized its role as the 'coordinating authority', putting itself in a privileged position vis-à-vis its partners and competitors.

In spite of the ridicule which the role of coordination met in some comments on the WHO's early response to Ebola, coordination is, in fact, one of the main roles of the WHO (see also Turshen and Tefera, 2017). According to the WHO Constitution, 'the functions of the Organization shall be: (a) to act as the directing and coordinating authority on international health work; (b) to establish and maintain effective collaboration with [other] organizations'.[11] But these are only two of more than twenty different functions. Other functions certainly grant the WHO responsibility over actual programmes and activities. As mentioned above, the WHO's reputation was gained when the Organization took upon itself ambitious, pro-active interventionist projects, such as the eradication of smallpox, and also when it took an adversarial position in emergency situations, as was the case with SARS, when Director-General Brundtland took what the *New York Times* reported to be an 'unusually aggressive stance', 'hectoring' the Chinese government to share more information about the disease. When the Chinese government did not cooperate, Dr Brundtland issued a global alert

(Flynn and Nebehay, 2014; Sengupta, 2015). Indeed, as the case of SARS shows, under Dr Brundtland's leadership the WHO bureaucracy seemed to have little interest in narrowing the scope of the Organization's responsibilities. Still, essays on the future of the WHO from the late 1990s indicate increasing sensitivity to the need to define a narrower role for the Organization that would avoid the need to compete with new health entities while still maintaining its leadership position – and 'coordination' was that role (see, for example, Yamey, 2002b).

Coordination also allowed the WHO to better adapt to a new fashionable concept, that of 'ownership'. The concept of 'ownership' or 'country ownership' – which was initially developed by the IMF and the World Bank (Branson and Hanna, 2000; Khan and Sharma, 2001; World Bank, 1999) – conventionally holds that 'countries themselves set their priorities, design programmes, implement them and are accountable for what is being achieved' (Kazatchkine, 2008). However, the principle of 'ownership' is quite foreign to and potentially incompatible with the governing logic of the WHO. While it respects country sovereignty in the form of equal participation – policies and programmes at the WHO are initiated, debated and decided at the international level – once those policies are decided, all countries are expected to accept and follow those policies. Sovereignty means that member states can tell the organization what to do. Not that the organization does not get to make decisions (see Chorev, Andia and Ciplet, 2014).

There is minimal, if any, strategic manipulation in the WHO's adhering to the narrowing implications of coordination and ownership. Nevertheless, under the leadership of Director-General Chan, as was the case with Ebola, the function of coordination and the principle of ownership were used as a way to lower expectations and to defend the WHO from potential criticism, given its limited capabilities.

To summarize, from the early 1990s the WHO's bureaucracy responded to neoliberal pressures by adopting policies that gave a new meaning to the neoliberal logic. For the most part, strategic adaptation allowed the WHO to save some of its preferences and interests. As I described above, by defining health 'in economic terms' the WHO was able to protect the relative prominence of health in international considerations; by accepting cost-effective logic it was able to legitimate interventions in the three major diseases killing the poor, including those that were not necessarily the most cost-effective; and by redefining its position it was able to insist on its leadership status in an increasingly crowded field without, at least in principle, having to get involved in projects that it did not have the capabilities to support.

But strategic adaptation does not come without cost. And the WHO's response to Ebola highlights some of the costs involved in compliance, even if it is strategic. The implications are important: if the failure to respond adequately to the Ebola crisis was the outcome of adaptive strategies, it means that the Ebola failure did not just happen. Rather, it was the result of decisions made by the WHO in order to remain relevant at all. In the next section I describe the historical context of the main factors leading to the WHO's initial response to Ebola, and draw on that historical context to evaluate the WHO's recent plans of organizational reform.

The costs of strategic adaptation

Two of the main issues on which commentators criticizing the WHO's response to the Ebola outbreak focused were budget constraints and the shifting of priorities away from communicable diseases. As we have seen, insufficient budgets, leading to the lack of adequate attention to the monitoring of outbreaks, are the outcome of significant structural transformations.

The pressure on the WHO to cut its budget was particularly heavy following the global financial crisis in 2008 – after which the WHO cut its already limited budget by 20% (Fink, 2014a) – but this was not an unprecedented event. Rather, the WHO has been under ongoing, relentless, sometimes quite assertive pressure to cut its budget since at least the early 1990s. This was partly a result of the growing mistrust in bureaucracies, particularly 'politicized' bureaucracies, to act efficiently or effectively. It was also a reflection of member states and other donors choosing, as described above, to support competing international health entities – including public-private partnerships. It is in this context of a particularly limited budget, and as part of the WHO's strategic embrace of cost-effective calculations, that the Organization shifted its priorities from communicable to non-communicable diseases, with some notable exceptions. Cost-effective calculations are likely to result in the prioritization of non-communicable diseases, such as diabetes or cancer, over communicable diseases, particularly one-time outbreaks, not only because at least some chronic diseases are considered easier to prevent and treat than many communicable diseases, but also because of the great difficulty in calculating outbreaks that are entirely unpredictable in their timing and likely cost.

The adoption of cost-effective calculations as the tool for setting the WHO's priorities, therefore, inevitably led to the neglect of outbreaks monitoring. In response to increasing budgetary constraints, the WHO cuts included an 8% cut in the funds devoted to infectious diseases and a remarkable 51% cut in the funds devoted to outbreak and crisis response, from $469 million to a mere $228 million (Butler, 2013). In turn, the WHO staff charged with emergency response was reduced from ninety-four people to thirty-four (Fink, 2014a). At the regional level, budget cuts forced the African office to cut its epidemic team from twelve to four (Flynn and Nebehay, 2014). (At the same time, there is a separate budget item that is devoted to helping countries to respond to outbreaks on their own, and that budget increased by 32% [Butler, 2013] – reflecting, no doubt, the new interest in ownership).

A disproportionate reliance on voluntary donations, even if these are less likely to closely follow priorities based on cost-effective calculations, also contributed to the diminishing availability of funds for outbreaks such as Ebola. Voluntary donations, which are 'earmarked' to projects of interest to the contributing nations, are more likely to be given to projects that capture the public imagination rather than to issues such as 'preparedness'. No doubt, voluntary donations were fundamental to the international response *once* the WHO had alerted its member states to the Ebola crisis. Still, even while recognizing the magnitude of the harm, donations were initially slow to come (Hicken, 2014), and these donations are mostly devoted to containing the current outbreak rather than preventing the next one. Such donations also often dry up as soon as the issue is no longer on the front pages of the *New York Times* and other newspapers. As Director-General Chan once complained, 'When there's an event, we have money. Then after that, the money stops coming in' (quoted in Fink, 2014b).

Commentators also had deep concerns regarding the WHO's insistence on a relatively narrow task of coordination and on countries' ownership. Hence, while criticizing the WHO's initial inability to achieve the goal of coordination effectively (Flynn and Nebehay, 2014), commentators also denounced the WHO's view and made it clear that they expected the Organization to 'quickly muster an army of experts and health workers to combat an outbreak overtaking some of the world's poorest countries' (Fink, 2014a).

In this debate, the WHO is correct. As I described above, coordination is indeed a central constitutional function of the WHO. But in the past a broader, more ambitious agenda allowed it to fail many times – including in its decades-long attempt to eradicate malaria – but also to succeed in ways that not only increased its reputation but, unintentionally, increased expectations regarding its actual abilities. However, combined with the concept of ownership, the WHO had little that it could coordinate, or even guide. Ownership is used most often by organizations – such as the Global Fund to Fight AIDS, Tuberculosis and Malaria – that engage in the distribution of generous grants. In response to criticisms of 'top-down' imposition of priorities and programmes, 'ownership' provided a way for such organizations to be more responsive to what countries need and want (Chorev, Andia and Ciplet, 2014). But the WHO is not such an organization – it does not have the means to distribute grants and it does not, therefore, have the means to ensure the state capacity that is required for 'ownership' to work. The International Health Regulations embed the concept of ownership by delegating some of the responsibilities for the monitoring of outbreaks from the WHO to member states; for that purpose, the Regulations also oblige countries to develop 'core public health capacities'. But, contributing to the inadequate response to Ebola and other health crises, by the deadline in 2012 only 20% of nations – and very few in Africa – had put in place the necessary regulations and programmes (Morgan, 2014).

Of course, the failure to follow the International Health Regulations is a symptom of the weak health infrastructure – as well as of regulatory capabilities – in many poor countries. And lack of health care infrastructure has particularly disastrous effects in moments of emergency, leading not only to the inability of governments to respond effectively but also to the utter collapse of the entire health system. As many public health experts have suggested, Ebola is, first and foremost, a symptom of a weak health care system (Farmer, 2014). The prevalence of inadequate health care systems in many poor countries has much to do with lack of domestic resources, but also with the WHO's and others' lack of investment in infrastructure. International programmes today tend to concentrate on immediate deliverables, such as insecticide-treated bed-nets or medicines, rather than on the building of health clinics or the training of health workers. The recent organizational fragmentation of international health activities – with the emergence of many new organizations, funds and partnerships – has also inadvertently contributed to the lack of investment in health infrastructure. Such fragmentation – where different organizations have responsibility for diverse specific goals – offers many advantages. The GAVI Alliance, for example, has been fundamental in improving access to vaccines. But such organizational cacophony and minute division of labour is particularly ill equipped to support local health systems, in turn weakening the possibility of effective coordination and ownership.

The criticisms directed at the WHO were severe and required a public response. At first, as we have seen, the WHO leadership was excessively defensive – illustrated most clearly in Dr Chan's remark that expectations of the WHO were a 'fantasy' (Fink, 2014a). But time allowed the WHO not only to contribute to operational activities in West Africa but also to alter its own thinking on the matter. For example, a Report of the Ebola Interim Assessment Panel,[12] commissioned by the WHO, led to a resolution at the World Health Assembly in May 2015 that committed the Organization to 'sweeping institutional reforms to bolster the agency's rapid response capacity' (Patrick, 2015).

It is useful to note that this resolution and other such steps were a response to an unprecedented crisis. In the past, the WHO had been the subject either of pointed criticisms regarding a specific programme, which required, at the most, local adjustments, or of overarching criticisms regarding the institution as a whole, as was the case in the late 1980s, which called for an overall transformation of the institution's identity – as happened, for example, under the leadership of Dr Brundtland. This time the WHO suffered from a pointed criticism, but with a level of severity that seemed to require nothing short of an overall transformation. Indeed, some commentators suggested that a reform 'could begin the long effort to restore the WHO's credibility and leadership in global public health' (Patrick, 2015). However, even if reforms improve the preparedness capabilities of the WHO and its member states, there is nothing that a targeted reform can do on its own to free the WHO from the constraints it has been facing since the 1990s. Reforms are necessarily focused on the task at hand – one suggestion, for example, was the creation of a reserve of public health workers, supported by a contingency fund.[13] Such plans might indeed improve the WHO's future response to outbreaks; but such plans accept rather than challenge the logic under which the WHO currently operates, and therefore cannot possibly improve its *overall* ability to respond to global health needs. The plan to have a reserve of public health workers, for example, relies on voluntary contributions and requires a voluntary commitment from countries not as member states but as donors. And many suggested reforms not only rely on 'partnerships with key UN agencies and other international responders', as Director-General Chan assured the World Health Assembly,[14] but also have to compete with alternative plans, such as the World Bank's suggested creation of a funding group for pandemics.[15] Put differently, while the WHO certainly has the capacity to have some programmes work well and to improve other programmes, any improvement is necessarily limited by the existing institutional and structural constraints and by the strategies used by the WHO in responding to them. Nothing in the response to the Ebola crisis of 2014–16 looked like the kind of institutional revolution that some commentators wanted. One could even more critically conclude that here, once again, the WHO was forced to respond to a popularity contest among different urgent programmes in a context of scarce resources, with outbreaks (momentarily) at the top of the list.

Conclusion

The immediate, most proximate and easily identifiable factors that led to the inadequacy of the WHO's initial response to the Ebola outbreak have historical, structural foundations. By identifying these structural factors we are able to see that the budget cuts, the de-prioritization of outbreak monitoring and the WHO's avoidance of operational assistance – but also its plans of organizational reform – were all part of a larger transformation, one that was triggered by the WHO's response to the neoliberal turn. Concretely, many of the conditions that impacted on the WHO's response can be traced back to the late 1990s and early 2000s, when its bureaucracy – facing authority, financial and legitimacy crises – was forced to respond to a changing world. Instead of either complying with or resisting neoliberal prescriptions, the WHO leadership manoeuvred external expectations in a way that allowed it to save many of the preferences and interests at the core of the Organization's mission. But such strategic manoeuvring did come with compromises and necessary costs, and the early response to Ebola puts into bald relief what the international community has lost by reducing its international health organization to a resource-poor 'coordinating' unit.

Significantly, coordination is central to the very influential argument regarding the move from 'international' to 'global' public health (Brown, Cueto and Fee, 2006). The classical pieces that attempt to define that move describe, first, the growing importance of additional actors in the international arena, and second, the ability of the WHO to maintain its leadership role precisely by functioning as a coordinator. Indeed, earlier on, Yach and Bettcher (1988) had already celebrated the potential of coordination by referring in particular to disease outbreaks. The WHO, they promised, 'could help create more efficient information and surveillance systems by strengthening its global monitoring and alert systems'. But the response to Ebola in 2014 might indicate that being 'global' – in the sense of reducing the WHO's role to that of coordination and leaving the bulk of responsibilities not only to countries with uneven capabilities but also to other international health organizations – does not work. It indicates that coordination requires capabilities and that capabilities, too, should be part of the global public health agenda.

Notes

1 This information draws on WHO Fact Sheet No. 103, www.who.int/mediacentre/factsheets/fs103/en/ (accessed 9 December 2015); Centers for Disease Control and Prevention report, https://www.cdc.gov/vhf/ebola/history/2014-2016-outbreak/index.html (accessed 18 October 2019).
2 See www.who.int/ihr/publications/9789241596664/en/ (accessed 9 December 2015).
3 See www.who.int/mediacentre/multimedia/Ebola_outbreak_Guinea_transcript_08APR2014.pdf (accessed 9 December 2015).
4 See www.msf.ca/en/article/ebola-west-africa-epidemic-out-control (accessed 9 December 2015).
5 See www.who.int/mediacentre/news/statements/2014/ebola-20140808/en/ (accessed 9 December 2015).
6 See www.who.int/csr/resources/publications/ebola/report-by-panel.pdf?ua=1 (accessed 9 December 2015).

7 Richard Brennan, director of the WHO's Department of Emergency Risk Management and Humanitarian Response, quoted in Sun et al. (2014).
8 This analysis relies in part on Chorev (2012a); see Abdullah and Rashid (2017) for a comprehensive consideration of Ebola in the neoliberal context.
9 See www.who.int/about/finances-accountability/funding/financing-dialogue/Programme-Budget-2016–2017-Prospectus.pdf (accessed 12 December 2015).
10 Other international initiatives, including the Millennium Development Goals (signed in 2000) and the Global Fund to Fight AIDS, Tuberculosis and Malaria (established in 2002) also focus on the same three diseases. This emerging international consensus was in part enabled by the WHO's earlier strategic response.
11 See www.who.int/governance/eb/who_constitution_en.pdf (accessed 12 December 2015).
12 See https://www.who.int/csr/resources/publications/ebola/report-by-panel.pdf?ua=1 (accessed 18 October 2019).
13 See http://apps.who.int/gb/ebwha/pdf_files/WHA68/A68_ACONF5-en.pdf (accessed 17 December 2015).
14 See www.who.int/dg/speeches/2015/68th-wha/en/ (accessed 17 December 2015).
15 See www.worldbank.org/en/topic/pandemics/brief/pandemic-emergency-facility-frequently-asked-questions (accessed 17 December 2015).

References

Abbasi, K. (1999) 'The World Bank and World Health: Changing Sides', *British Medical Journal* 318 (7187), 865–869.

Abdullah, Ibrahim and Ismail Rashid (eds) (2017) *Understanding West Africa's Ebola Epidemic: Towards a Political Economy*. London: Zed Books.

Babb, S. (2009) *Behind the Development Banks*. Chicago, IL: University of Chicago Press.

Birmingham, K. (1999) 'Brundtland Makes Waves in Her First Six Months at the WHO', *Nature Medicine* 5 (3), 249.

Branson, W. and Nagy Hanna (2000) 'Ownership and Conditionality', *Operations Evaluation Department (OED) Working Paper Series*. Washington, DC: World Bank.

Brenner, N. and N. Theodore (2002) 'Cities and the Geographies of "Actually Existing Neoliberalism"', *Antipode* 34 (3), 356–386.

Brown, T. M., M. Cueto, and E. Fee (2006) 'The World Health Organization and the Transition from "International" to "Global" Public Health', *American Journal of Public Health* 96 (1), 62–72.

Brundtland, Gro Harlem (2000) 'Speech at the Opening of the Third Meeting of the Commission for Macroeconomics and Health', Third Meeting of the Commission on Macroeconomics and Health. Paris.

Butler, D. (2013) 'Agency Gets a Grip on Budget', *Nature* 498 (7452), 6 June, 18–19.

Chorev, N. (2012a) *The World Health Organization between North and South*. Ithaca, NY: Cornell University Press.

Chorev, N. (2012b) 'Changing Global Norms through Reactive Diffusion: The Case of Intellectual Property Protection of AIDS Drugs', *American Sociological Review* 77 (5), 831–853.

Chorev, N., T. Andia and D. Ciplet (2014) 'The State of States in International Organizations', *Review* 34 (3), 285–310.

CMH (Commission on Macroeconomics and Health) (2001) *Macroeconomics and Health: Investing in Health for Economic Development*. Geneva: World Health Organization.

Cox, R. W. (1986) *Production, Power and World Order*. New York: Columbia University Press.

Farmer, P. (2014) 'Diary', *London Review of Books* 36 (20), 38–39.

Fink, S. (2014a) 'Cuts at W.H.O. Hurt Response to Ebola Crisis', *New York Times*, 3 September.

Fink, S. (2014b) 'W.H.O. Leader Describes the Agency's Ebola Operations', *New York Times*, 4 September.

Flynn, D. and S. Nebehay (2014) 'Aid Workers Ask Where Was WHO in Ebola Outbreak?' *Reuters*, October 6.

Godlee, F. (1994a) 'WHO in Crisis', *British Medical Journal* 309 (6966), 1424–1428.

Godlee, F. (1994b) 'WHO in Retreat: Is It Losing Its Influence?' *British Medical Journal* 309 (6967), 1491–1495.

Harvey, D. (2005) *A Brief History of Neoliberalism*. New York: Oxford University Press.

Hicken, M. (2014) 'Ebola Donations Lag Far Behind Need', CNN, 8 October.

Kazatchkine, M. (2008) Blog-interview at *The Herald Tribune*, 12 March, www.eatg.org/news/163686/Q_%26_A_with_Michel_Kazatchkine_of_The_Global_Fund.

Khan, M. S. and Sunil Sharma (2001) 'IMF Conditionality and Country Ownership of Programs', *IMF Working Paper*, WP/01/142. International Monetary Fund (IMF) Institute, www.imf.org/external/pubs/ft/wp/2001/wp01142.pdf.

Lee, K. (2009) *The World Health Organization (WHO)*. London: Routledge.
Lee, K. and Gill Walt (1992) 'What Role for WHO in the 1990s?' *Health Policy and Planning* 7 (4), 387–390.
Morgan, D. (2014) 'U.S. Says Diseases Like Ebola Should Be Viewed As Security Threats', *Reuters*, 26 September.
New York Times Editorial Board (2014) 'A Painfully Slow Ebola Response', *New York Times*, 15 August.
Oliver, C. (1991) 'Strategic Responses to Institutional Pressures', *Academy of Management Review* 16 (1), 145–79.
Packard, R. M. (2009) '"Roll Back Malaria, Roll in Development"? Reassessing the Economic Burden of Malaria', *Population and Development Review* 35 (1), 53–87.
Park, A. (2014) 'Why the World Health Organization Doesn't Have Enough Funds to Fight Ebola', *Mother Jones*, 8 September.
Patrick, S. M. (2015) 'Course Correction: WHO Reform after Ebola', Blog. *Council for Foreign Relations*, 27 January, http://blogs.cfr.org/patrick/2015/01/27/course-correction-who-reform-after-ebola/.
Renwick, D. and T. Johnson (2014) 'The World Health Organization (WHO)', *CFR Backgrounders*. Council on Foreign Relations, 7 October, www.cfr.org/public-health-threats-and-pandemics/world-health-organization-/p20003.
Richter, J. (2004) 'Public-Private Partnerships for Health: A Trend with No Alternatives?', *Development* 47 (2), 43–48.
Sack, K., S. Fink, P. Belluck and A. Nossiter (2014) 'How Ebola Roared Back', *New York Times*, 29 December.
Sengupta, S. (2015) 'Effort on Ebola Hurt W.H.O. Chief', *New York Times*, 6 January.
Sun, L., B. Dennis, L. Bernstein, and J. Achenba (2014) 'Out of Control: How the World's Health Organizations Failed to Stop the Ebola Disaster', *Washington Post*, 4 October.
Turshen, Meredeth and Gezmu Tefera (2017) 'The World Health Organization and the Ebola Epidemic', in *Understanding West Africa's Ebola Epidemic: Towards a Political Economy*, ed. Ibrahim Abdullah and Ismail Rashid (pp. 244–262). London: Zed Books.
Walt, G. and K. Buse (2000) 'Editorial: Partnership and Fragmentation in International Health: Threat or Opportunity?', *Tropical Medicine and International Health* 5 (7), 467–471.
Walt, G., Neil Spicer, and Ken Buse (2009) 'Mapping the Global Health Architecture', in *Making Sense of Global Health Governance: A Policy Perspective*, ed. K. Buse, W. Hein and N. Drager (pp. 47–71). Houndmills: Palgrave Macmillan.

World Bank (1993) *World Development Report: Investing in Health*, Washington, DC: IBRD.
World Bank (1999) *Higher Impact Adjustment Lending (HIAL): Initial Evaluation, vol. 1*. Operations Evaluation Department, Report No. 19797. Washington, DC: World Bank, http://ieg.assyst-uc.com/Data/reports/hial.pdf.
WHO (2000) *World Health Report 2000. Health Systems: Improving Performance*. Geneva: WHO.
Yach, D. and D. Bettcher (1988) 'The Globalisation of Public Health', *American Journal of Public Health*, 88, 735–741.
Yamey, G. (2002a) 'WHO in 2002: Interview with Gro Brundtland', *British Medical Journal* 325 (7376), 1355–1358.
Yamey, G. (2002b) 'WHO in 2002: Why Does the World Still Need WHO?', *British Medical Journal* 325 (7375), 1294–1298.

10

Epilogue: in search of global health

Didier Fassin

Prologue

For anyone who thinks of global health in the mid-2010s, the event that immediately and spontaneously comes to mind is the 2014 Ebola epidemic. It was described as a 'global crisis' by Harvard Medical School, called a 'global security threat' by the president of the US and declared a 'global health emergency' by the WHO. Yet, the question that can be posed is: how global was the epidemic? Or perhaps more accurately: what was global in the epidemic? And in what sense was it global? In a direct and probably too simple way, I propose the following answer to these questions: the outbreak was mostly local and partially regional; the response was essentially national and somewhat international; only the representation and the consequent affects were global.

First, the feared outbreak was confined to three countries – Sierra Leone, Liberia and, to a lesser degree, Guinea – where 99.8% of the 11,000 deaths were concentrated, and although the virus was spread in these countries, almost all cases were in a limited number of villages and towns; there were only six cases outside of sub-Saharan Africa, with one death, representing 0.01% of the total. Second, the much-criticized response on the ground was principally that of the impoverished and deficient national health systems, whose professionals paid a high toll in terms of the epidemic's lethality; and it benefited from the assistance of international NGOs, particularly Médecins sans Frontières, whose engagement was widely celebrated. By contrast, as Nitsan

Chorev discusses in chapter 9 of this volume, the WHO was accused of not taking the epidemic seriously enough at its inception, although this relatively unfair criticism can be viewed in retrospect as the effect of an exaggerated assessment of the outbreak. As for the assistance of nations from the rest of the world, the most spectacular effort was that of the US, which sent 3,000 troops and created twenty clinical facilities in the region to treat 28 of the 28,000 Ebola patients, half of the medical centres having received not a single case. Third, the idea of a worldwide threat and the resulting fear were global in a way that was out of proportion with the reality of the risk and led to excessive populist reactions from certain political leaders. A US opinion poll in November 2014 showed that Ebola came in third position among the most urgent health problems facing the country, just after cost and access, but ahead of cancer and heart diseases, which account for half the deaths in the US, and that almost one in two persons interviewed were worried that either they or one of their relatives would become sick with Ebola. And while CNN, NBC and CBS were devoting hours of breaking news to the cases of a physician and a nurse who had returned from the region, actively contributing to producing fear and misrepresentations, the governors of the states of New York and New Jersey decided to quarantine health workers coming back from areas where the virus was prevalent, against the recommendations of the Centers for Disease Control (CDC) and the National Institute of Infectious Diseases, which came under heavy media pressure for not doing enough. Referring to her experience with the H1N1 influenza vaccination in the US, Danielle Ofri (2009) had called in the *New England Journal of Medicine* for an 'emotional epidemiology' of emergent infectious diseases, while in the *Journal of Infectious Diseases* Daniel Bausch and Marguerite Clougherty (2015) questioned the 'sensationalist bent' that had surrounded the Ebola epidemic.

In sum, there was no global viral epidemic. The global crisis was emotional, the global threat was fantasized, the global emergency was hyperbolized. If there was a global epidemic, it was of representations and affects. In articulating these straightforward statements I am not trying to express any form of critical judgement on human actions and reactions in the face of the epidemic, which are ultimately not so different from what they have been in previous, similar events. I am simply attempting to re-evaluate the various dimensions of a phenomenon commonly thought of as global. One could retort that it is easier to make such an assessment a posteriori than a priori. This is true, and obviously so of all our studies, historical or not: our analyses are always ex post – although I should add, without claiming any merit for it, that, when I was consulted, I foretold, on the basis of the low contagiosity of the infection and the experience of previous outbreaks (my very first internship in infectious diseases in the 1980s was in the only hospital in France which had a special section for Ebola cases), a limited expansion of the epidemic at the very moment when some experts at the CDC were talking of possibly more than one million cases. Of course, it could be argued that the global fear contributed to the international response, which strengthened the national responses and therefore contained the spreading of the virus – an optimistic interpretation of the role of human intervention which few epidemiologists would support. But my point is neither to minimize the potential risks of such epidemics and the unavoidable uncertainty about such risks nor to lambast the overreaction of some, in contrast with the slow response of others, probably involving in both cases strategic intentions, notably to mobilize aid in the first case and to play down the situation in the second.

My argument is twofold. First, it is crucial to differentiate several facets of what is called global health: are we talking about a disease, the management of a disease or the representation of a disease? These aspects are often confused or considered to evolve alongside one another. The Ebola case suggests that more analytical caution is necessary. Second, it is important to resist the form of hype that often accompanies the idea of global health, with its images of responsiveness and solidarity: diseases and their management remain largely local and national issues; international mobilization generally becomes possible when global concerns affect rich nations, whose members begin to fear for their own security. There is no stronger incentive to aid than the perceived danger to oneself. The Ebola case attests to a connectedness within the world community where benevolence is ultimately legitimized by self-interest. In other words, the Ebola story invites us to complicate our comprehension of global health by emphasizing, differentiating and relating its theoretical and moral dimensions.

Introduction

From this dual perspective, one could assert that global health as a notion or as a field is perhaps both under-conceptualized and over-normative, the two being linked (Fassin, 2012). On the one hand, the notion is often taken for granted, with little reference to the intense debates since the turn of the century with regard to globalization in the social and economic sciences, as if it simply described a novel phenomenon – although what is different from the previous state of public health in the world remains unclear. 'There is no common understanding of the term global health, agreement about the content of global health courses, or of what it means to work or conduct research on global health,' complain Sarah MacFarlane, Marian Jacobs and Ephata Kaaya (2008) in an essay on the topic. On the other hand, the field is saturated by the noble objective of improving public health in the world, and social scientists are invited, or invite themselves, to the table so long as they can participate in its accomplishment. 'The ultimate goal of anthropological work in and of global health is to reduce global health inequities and contribute to the development of sustainable and salutogenic sociocultural, political, and economic systems,' assert Craig Janes and Kitty Corbett (2009) in their review of the literature on the subject. Thus, when considering the rapid multiplication of academic programmes and philanthropic institutions under the name 'global health', especially in the US, one would be tempted to think that the cart of the catchword has been put before the horse of the concept.

There might be good reasons for that: a sense of urgency – the problems of a suffering humanity cannot wait. But urgency to do what? To 'repair the world', to quote a title from one of our most famous global health scholars, or to label a new domain in order to attract interest and funding, while doing more or less the same thing? It is well known that this was the reason why the WHO changed its orientation from the old-fashioned international health to the more trendy global health, as Theodore Brown, Marcos Cueto and Elizabeth Fee (2006) convincingly argued: the same programmes under another name at a time when private charities, such as the Bill and Melinda Gates Foundation, had become major players in the field under the new banner. And there is certainly nothing to be criticized in this rebranding of activities and institutions to make them more attractive to their publics or donors. The academic and philanthropic worlds function as markets, after all, and not only in the US: they have to sell their products. But this should not be a sufficient reason to avoid an analytical approach and a critical reflection. From this perspective, rather than discussing a definition – an exercise of limited value – I will propose five lines of tension which underlie the domain of global health.

These lines of tension allow for an understanding of global health as a social field of political, economic, symbolic and cognitive forces. They crystallize a series of issues and stakes that are all related to the unequal state of the world – not only in terms of morbidity, mortality, life expectancy, physical well-being, but also in terms of resources, knowledge, rights, morality. This global inequality often has a sort of verticality – the North versus the South – although it can also be regarded as horizontal – the West versus the Rest, an expression which I prefer to use in the company of Stuart Hall rather than of Niall Ferguson.

Tension 1: worldwide versus universal

The adjective 'global' suggests a dual type of expansion – spatial and ideological. As a spatial descriptor it means worldwide: it implies interconnectedness beyond national borders, whether that concerns the dissemination of viruses or habits, the circulation of people or money, the flows of technologies or drugs. As an ideological descriptor, it means universal: it signifies a claim to certain truths, whether they have to do with epistemological models, political choices, ethical values. Policies of control may be implemented in the first case to limit the propagation of microbes, the movements of population or the introduction of certain medicines. Politics of domination may be involved in the second case to impose paradigms, programmes or priorities. The two aspects are often confused and the worldwide slogan tends to become a universalist claim.

The HIV epidemic is a case in point for these epistemological, political and ethical predicaments. Thus, during its first two decades, and even beyond, the epidemiological interpretation of the rapid spread of the infection on the African continent was exclusively focused on sexual behaviour, sexual promiscuity and sexual violence, often at the cost of racist extrapolations, as Gilles Bibeau (1991) showed. By contrast, the social causes leading to survival sex and the medical responsibilities related to unsafe injections were systematically ignored. Similarly, the President's Emergency Plan for AIDS Relief, PEPFAR, which its promoters claimed to be the most important health initiative ever taken by a single country, was, especially during the first years of its existence, heavily inscribed in a political agenda with moral implications, imposing abstinence until marriage, rejecting prevention in the case of sex workers, excluding needle-exchange programmes for drug addicts and privileging collaboration with faith-based organizations. Beyond these specific issues, the plan implied a form of intervention on populations which Vinh-Kim Nguyen (2009) named 'government-by-exception'. Finally, the design of actions for poor countries involved ethical questions which were left unaddressed or subsequently corrected in contradictory ways, as was denounced by Marcia Angell (1997) in a review of a series of clinical trials to prevent mother-to-child transmission. Initially, these interventions, conceived to avoid the infection of children at birth and during their first months of life, did not include the treatment of mothers and even did not consider the risk of drug resistance, which jeopardized future multi-therapy (Fassin, 2015). Then, two successive protocols relying on opposing ethics were implemented in Africa. According to the first, minimalist ethic, nevirapine, presented as a magic bullet, was the cheap solution best adapted to poor countries, which led to overlooking its negative side-effects. According to the second, maximalist ethic, the same modality had to be applied as in rich countries, at whatever cost. In these various examples – epistemological, political and ethical – more than the errors, prejudices and hesitations, it is the way they are imposed each time, with the same hubris, under the argument of emergency, that is problematic.

Indeed, the assertive tone and frequently authoritarian approach to global health challenge both state sovereignty and national independence in the countries where these programmes are conducted through apparently neutral and depoliticized apparatuses which James Ferguson (1994) analyses as an 'anti-politics machine'. They provoke negative reactions from governments, sometimes from scientists and often from the public. These reactions can go from denial to opposition, from hidden resentment to open contestation, from rejecting the idea of an African origin of the virus to imagining an importation of the disease by Westerners – a remarkable illustration of the variety of ways of resisting symbolic or political domination with the 'weapons of the weak' as James Scott (1985) designates them. Such was the case in the first decades of the HIV epidemic, when interpretations of the infection, nourished by post-colonial prejudices and programmes of prevention inspired by neo-colonial practices, produced a counter-reaction that rendered discourses about and policies against AIDS ineffective for a long time. But local responses may also take an opposite form, that of mimicking, which inspired Homi Bhabba's (1994) reflections on post-coloniality. Such is the case with the adoption of procedures resembling clinical trials or medical experiments by local healers – usually the least traditional and the most charlatan among them – to validate their alleged miracle treatment of HIV infections.

Tension 2: moral versus economic

The noun 'health' refers to two sorts of realities – moral and economic. On the moral side, health has come to be viewed as a common good that must be protected: hence the various forms of social security, medical assistance, humanitarian aid, to guarantee access to health care; hence the legitimacy of mandatory measures to protect the health of the population such as the treatment and isolation of contagious patients. On the economic side, health is also a commoditized good that has an increasing place in markets: hence the development of patenting and re-patenting for drugs and tests; hence the extraordinary profits of the pharmaceutical industry as well as insurance companies. Tensions between health as common good and health as commoditized good constantly arise.

One of the fiercest battles has been around the Affordable Care Act, also known as Obamacare, to expand the right to health care to twenty million people in the US, but the vehemence of the debate has left no space to discuss the extremely poor performance of the health care system as such in terms of its impact on the health of the population: it is probably the least cost-effective in the world. Another one – perhaps even more epic – was the 2001 Doha Round, which followed the 1994 Trade-Related Aspects of Intellectual Property Rights (TRIPS) Agreement of the World Trade Organization and made medicines in developing countries an exception to the general neoliberal move toward the protection of intellectual property; an exception contested, however, by

In search of global health

the US, which has since then been renegotiating multiple bilateral agreements, as shown by Gaëlle Krikorian (2014) for Morocco and Thailand. Obamacare was a national battle, the Doha Round a global one. A hybrid case was the 2001 Pretoria trial, when thirty-nine major pharmaceutical companies withdrew their complaint against the South African government, which considered that public health should prevail over intellectual property: this was the result of a successful collaboration between the Treatment Action Campaign and NGOs such as Act-Up and Médecins sans Frontières, in other words, between national and international actors. This paved the way for what Maurice Cassier (2008) called a 'new drug geopolitics', and it was both a national affair and a global endeavour.

But health itself is not a self-contained notion that can be defined once and for all, either as a common good or as a commoditized good, or both. It continually expands to include new aspects of human life. Through lead poisoning, characterized by Gerald Markowitz and David Rosner (2014) as 'lead wars', health relates to dilapidated housing for the poor as well as industrial contamination in disadvantaged neighbourhoods (Fassin, 2004). Through the pathologies of the poor, problematized by Paul Farmer (2004) in terms of 'structural violence', health addresses the issues of inequalities, which involve the distribution of wealth and the politics of social justice (Fassin, 2003). Through the post-traumatic stress disorder, analysed by Allan Young (1997), and child abuse, studied by Barbara Nelson (1984), the question of violence enters the domain of health (Fassin and Rechtman, 2009). Thus, not only is the territory of what we consider health to be in constant expansion but health has become the last language to address complex social issues legitimately and consensually, sometimes with the ultimate justification of contributing to the security of the world.

Tension 3: compassion versus predation

The translation of global health into concrete programmes realizes a peculiar mix of compassion and predation – compassion being generally on the medical side and predation on the scientific side. This is obviously not an absolute rule. Predatory medicine does exist: Nancy Scheper-Hughes's (2000) work on the global traffic of organs, from Brazil and South Africa to India and China for the givers, from the US to Israel for the receivers, leaves no doubt about that. And science can also prove to be compassionate: the Drugs for Neglected Diseases Initiative, which has been studied by Peter Redfield (2013), brings together the public sector, private companies and non-governmental actors to develop new treatments for pathologies whose medicines are non-profitable, such as sleeping sickness.

On the compassionate side, providing assistance to developing nations and impoverished populations confronted by dire needs, terrible famines, dreadful epidemics or ruinous disasters is a profound motivation for aid, the most characteristic form of which is humanitarian intervention conducted by states, international agencies or NGOs. Such action, the legitimization of which relies first and foremost on a sense of urgency, has received a lot of scholarly attention from political scientists such as Michael Barnett (2011). Beyond this specific type of undertaking, sometimes associated with military operations, medical assistance to Third World countries often combines sentiments of empathy and ideas of solidarity toward the sick and the poor. Yet it reflects the moral priorities of the helper rather than the practical priorities of the helped. During the first decades of the HIV epidemic resentment among public health experts and government officials in developing countries toward the good will of UNAIDS and the numerous agencies proposing or imposing their aid frequently resulted from their conviction that more pressing problems, which had long been neglected, were still being ignored, such as acute respiratory infections, diarrhoea and measles. I remember in the late 1980s leading a well-endowed mission for the European Union in Peru, where the country's only AIDS patient was isolated in a special unit, while major poverty-related diseases were regarded by my interlocutors as much more serious issues. Even today this remains the case, as was shown by Julie Livingston (2012) in her description of the only oncology ward in Botswana, which is underfunded and overcrowded, when the efforts of the international medical community are principally concentrated on HIV prevention and treatment.

On the other hand, the work of scientists in general and of life scientists in particular in poor countries or poor communities often consists in a form of extraction, when it is not sheer exploitation. Researchers come, collect their data, leave, publish their papers and come again for the next cycle. When the data are made of blood samples, as is often the case with clinical trials, the procedure resembles a form of international vampirism which is legitimized by the supposed benefits to the population. An extreme case of this predation is a University of California, Los Angeles multimillion-dollar programme which proposes to identify and prevent potential emergent retroviral diseases in animals before they get to humans. This initiative, which has benefited not only from huge funding from the National Institutes of Health but also from wide media coverage beyond the US, seems like a biological version of the film *Minority Report*, and is analysed by Guillaume Lachenal (2014) as a sort of nihilism that associates the grandeur of a celebrated science and the misery of an impotent medicine, a contrast which is derided by local commentators. Beyond this somewhat extravagant project, the Third World, and particularly the African continent, has become an attractive space in which to carry out biological investigations, experimental medicine and, notably, clinical trials, as is argued by Fanny Chabrol (2014), who speaks of a 'field of opportunities' for research teams from the North who can conduct their programmes at little cost, with minimal ethical constraints, with docile captive patients, sometimes even with the justification and satisfaction of providing free treatments to patients through these studies. This is what Adriana Petryna (2002) calls 'globalizing human subjects research'. Certainly building a scientific domain by using the biological and pathological material available in the South is hardly new, and in the late nineteenth and early twentieth century the Pasteur Institutes, studied by Anne-Marie Moulin (1992), constructed the field of tropical medicine via their presence in the colonial world and exploitation of local resources.

Tension 4: facts versus representations

A tension exists at the cognitive level – between facts and representations. On the side of science and medicine, which are largely generated in the North, even when they are destined for the South, it is considered that the knowledge which researchers and physicians produce is made of facts, which are real: they can be verified or falsified, according to their epistemology, through observation and experimentation. Evidence-based science, or medicine, and more recently public health, are the last avatars of this empiricist trend. Scientific and medical journals, conferences, networks validate and transmit this orthodox knowledge.

On the side of local populations, especially in the South but sometimes also in the North, the cognitive production is generally referred to in terms of beliefs in common parlance, mentalities in ancient ethnology or representations in modern anthropology. Whatever noun is used, and whatever effort is made to avoid the condescension attached to it, this form of knowledge is regarded as an illusion or a misconception. It is erroneous even if some well-intentioned social scientists affirm that it must be considered and even studied. In sum, facts exist in the material world, being objects of observation and experimentation, whereas representations exist in the imaginary world, being objects of description and interpretation. This common and comfortable differentiation, even when mitigated by an effort to be the most respectful of otherness, does not stand up to the test of critical analysis.

It is well known that facts themselves are constructed in a way that renders certain realities visible and others obscured. As Randall Packard (1989) demonstrated in the case of TB in South Africa during the first half of the twentieth century, biological theories focusing on genetic vulnerability and cultural interpretations emphasizing idiosyncratic behaviours were developed at the expense of the political economy of the disease. When I participated in the panel that was supposed to write the recommendations that UNAIDS would provide to ministers of health worldwide as guidelines for action against the HIV epidemic in the coming decade, it became clear at some point that technological solutions would definitely be privileged over social and political propositions: new tests for more precocious diagnosis of the infection over promotion of gender equality; techniques easily assessed through quantitative methods over practices accessible via qualitative approaches. Indeed, the major problem and even danger of evidence-based global health is that it gives consideration only to what can be measured rather than to what is relevant and significant, thus resembling the proverbial drunkard searching under the streetlight for the keys he has lost in the nearby park because it is the only place where there is light and where he can see.

But representations themselves are more than fantasies. Not only do they exist as social elements that contribute to the way social worlds are viewed and may ultimately be transformed, but they can also provide unexpected and overlooked truths. Conspiracy theories are interesting in this regard because they are generally presented and even derided as the most irrational and ridiculous representations (Fassin, 2011). They have multiplied since the mid-twentieth century about various issues, from Kennedy's assassination to the 9/11 attacks, but the domain of health has been particularly rich in such heterodox interpretations. These conspiracy theories may deserve more interest than is usually the case. In Ecuador, during the 1991 epidemic of cholera, indigenous people in the Andes fled from their villages as teams from the ministry of health arrived to screen, isolate and treat those infected: they remembered how the sick who had been taken to the hospital during a previous outbreak had died there alone, without the possibility for their families to visit them or even get the corpses back. In Nigeria the rejection of the polio vaccination programme implemented by the WHO in 2003 was interpreted as a sign of the backwardness of local Muslim religious leaders: however, this initiative followed a 1996 clinical trial in the same region of a new drug called Trovan and prescribed for meningitis which was considered to be the cause of numerous deaths and neurological complications, leading to its subsequent banning in Europe. The best-known case was in South Africa, where not only were dissenting interpretations of AIDS proposed at the highest level of the state from 2000 onwards, but rumours of a plot against the black population spread among the population as well as among decision makers. Actually, what Maynard Swanson (1977) termed the 'sanitation syndrome' had consisted, since the 1900 bubonic plague, in governments using the fear of infectious diseases, including influenza, syphilis and TB, to implement increasingly strict segregation rules and remove the black population from the urban areas to so-called native locations, later called townships. Thus, even in the apparently least defensible representations – that is, in conspiracy theories – something can be learned about real facts pertaining to the real world.

Tension 5: scale versus time

To end with a few methodological considerations, two oppositions seem to structure the approach of global health – one has to do with scale, the other with time. The question of scale is internal to the social sciences: the challenge is the connection between the micro of fieldwork and the macro of analysis. The question of time reaches outside of the social sciences: the challenge is the relation between the temporality of research and the temporality of action.

In her review of one of the first books on global health, Susan Glover (2009), after having underlined the qualities of the case studies presented in the volume, expressed her perplexity about how to move from these ethnographies of folk perceptions of disease to what she called a 'more cohesive theoretical perspective' on global health. This is a constant dilemma for medical anthropologists. How to remain faithful to one's situated findings while attempting to account for the larger picture? How to reach the global while staying local? There are various ways of solving this problem. One is a comparative design constructing a parallel between different worlds, as Margaret Lock (1993) does when she contrasts the local biologies of menopauses in Japan and North America to undermine the idea of a universal experience of physiological phenomena. Another is the multi-sited approach of interconnected scenes as presented by George Marcus (1995) in opposition to the traditional one-site approach in ethnography. Still another is the extended-case method inherited from Max Gluckman (1961) and later developed by Michael Burawoy (1998), consisting in relating local facts to the global scene, which would allow one to understand, for instance, the production of South African sites of high exposure to HIV for miners and women living near the mines within the broader context of the global mining industry. So much for scale.

But time is also a methodological issue. Global health is often associated with an idea of urgency, whether it is related to the fear of an epidemic that could become a pandemic, as in the case of H1N1 influenza or swine flu in Mexico, and H5N1 influenza or avian flu in China; or to the development of a humanitarian crisis in relation with a disaster or a conflict, as in Syria and Congo. By contrast, the social sciences, in particular those using ethnography, are criticized for their slowness, the months and years spent before being able to produce an informed description and a relevant interpretation: 'your findings come too late' is a comment frequently heard. This imputation can be discussed on two symmetrical grounds. First, what is claimed to be urgent often becomes chronic: the HIV epidemic has been described as an emergency for four decades and this has been an argument used against long-term research as opposed to quick methods such as RAP (rapid assessment programmes) or KABP (knowledge, attitude, beliefs and practices) surveys; in-depth enquiry surely deserve more consideration. Second, the duration of ethnographic studies is often compensated for by the fact that ethnographers, because their work is rarely motivated by the occurrence of events, as would be the case for journalists, are already there when these events happen; in other words, their presence can be viewed as early rather than late. These tensions between the temporalities of research and action must therefore be negotiated.

Conclusion

Most writings about global health present it as a desirable goal, attainable in a consensual way through scientific and moral progress, that is, as a result of expanded knowledge and increased solidarity. This is what the programme Solve at the Massachusetts Institute of Technology is about. Although I do not disregard these various dimensions and ambitions of global health, they are more on the prescriptive than the descriptive side: what it should be rather than what it is. I have tried instead to bring a less normative – or more realistic – view. The five lines of tensions – global as worldwide and universal, health as common good and commoditized good, global health action between compassion and predation, global health knowledge between facts and representations, global health methodology as a question of scale and time – suggest a social space of competition and struggle rather than a smooth linear path toward the well-being of the world. Global health is made of conflictive views and rival paradigms, of private interests and public goods, of scientific uncertainties and conspiracy theories, of practices of avoidance and discourses of resistance. Acknowledging these tensions and illuminating these contradictions, rather than attempting to ignore, deny or even resolve them, might be the most crucial task for social scientists.

References

Angell, M. (1997) 'The Ethics of Clinical Research in the Third World', *New England Journal of Medicine* 337, 847–849.

Barnett, M. (2011) *Empire of Humanity. A History of Humanitarianism*. New York: Cornell University Press.

Bausch, D. and M. Clougherty (2015) 'Ebola Virus: Sensationalism, Science, and Human Rights', *The Journal of Infectious Diseases* 212, S79–S83.

Bhabha, H. (1994) *The Location of Culture*. London: Routledge.

Bibeau, G. (1991) 'L'Afrique, terre imaginaire du sida. La subversion du discours scientifique par le jeu des fantasmes', *Anthropologie et Sociétés*, 15 (2–3), 125–147.

Brown, T., M. Cueto and E. Fee (2006) 'The World Health Organization and the Transition from "International" to "Global" Public Health', *American Journal of Public Health* 96 (1), 62–72.

Burawoy, M. (1998) 'The Extended Case Method', *Sociological Theory* 16 (1), 4–33.

Cassier, M. (2008) 'Une nouvelle géopolitique du medicament (1980–2005)', in *Des épidémies et des hommes*, ed. A. Flahault and P. Zylberman (pp. 101–109). Paris: la Martinière.

Chabrol, F. (2014) *Prendre soin de sa population. L'exception botswanaise face au sida*. Paris: Maison des Sciences de l'Homme.

Farmer, P. (2004) 'An Anthropology of Structural Violence', *Current Anthropology* 45 (3), 305–325.

Fassin, D. (2003) 'The Embodiment of Inequality. AIDS as a Social Condition and Historical Experience in South Africa', *Embo Reports*, 4, S4–S9.

Fassin, D. (2004) 'Public Health as Culture. The Social Construction of the Childhood Lead Poisoning Epidemic in France', *British Medical Bulletin*, 167–177, 691.

Fassin, D. (2011) 'The Politics of Conspiracy Theories. On AIDS in South Africa and a Few Other Global Plots', *The Brown Journal of World Affairs* 17 (2), 39–50.

Fassin, D. (2012) 'That Obscure Object of Global Health', in *Medical Anthropology at the Intersections. Histories, Activisms, and Futures*, ed. Marcia C. Inhorn and Emily A. Wentzell (pp. 95–115). Durham, NC: Duke University Press.

Fassin, D. (2015) 'Adventures of African Nevirapine. The Political Biography of a Magic Bullet', in *Para-States and Medical Science. Making African Global Health*, ed. Paul Wenzel Geissler (pp. 333–353). Durham NC: Duke University Press.

Fassin, D. and R. Rechtman (2009) *The Empire of Trauma: An Inquiry into the Condition of Victimhood*, trans. R. Gomme. Princeton, NJ: Princeton University Press.

Ferguson, J. (1994) *The Anti-Politics Machine. 'Development', Depoliticization, and Bureaucratic Power in Lesotho*. Minneapolis: University of Minnesota Press.

Glover, S. (2009) 'Review of "Mark Nichter: Global Health: Why Cultural Perceptions, Social Representations, and Biopolitics Matter"', *Human Ecology*, 37 (5), 669–670.

Gluckman, M. (1961) 'Ethnographic Data in British Social Anthropology', *The Sociological Review* 5–17, 91.
Janes, C. and K. Corbett (2009) 'Anthropology and Global Health', *Annual Review of Anthropology* 38, 167–183.
Krikorian, G. (2014) 'La propriété ou la vie? Économies morales, actions collectives et politiques du medicament dans la négociation d'accord de libre échange: Maroc, Thaïlande, États-Unis', Ph.D. dissertation, Paris: EHESS.
Lachenal, G. (2014) *Le médicament qui devait sauver l'Afrique. Un scandale pharmaceutique aux colonies.* Paris: La Découverte.
Livingston, J. (2012) *Improvising Medicine. An African Oncology Ward in an Emerging Cancer Epidemic.* Durham, NC: Duke University Press.
Lock, M. (1993) *Encounters with Aging. Mythologies of Menopause in Japan and North America.* Berkeley: University of California Press.
MacFarlane, S., M. Jacobs and Ephata Kaaya (2008) 'In the Name of Global Health: Trends in Academic Institutions', *Journal of Public Health Policy* 29, 383–401.
Marcus, G. (1995) 'Ethnography in/of the World System. The Emergence of Multi-Sited Ethnography', *Annual Review of Anthropology* 24, 95–117.
Markowitz, G. and D. Rosner (2014) *Lead Wars. The Politics of Science and the Fate of America's Children.* Berkeley: University of California Press.
Moulin, A.M. (1992) 'Patriarchal Science: The Network of the Overseas Pasteur Institutes', in *Science and Empires. Historical Studies about Scientific Development and European Expansion*, ed. P. Petitjean, C. Jami and Anne-Marie Moulin (pp. 307–322). Boston: Kluwer.
Nelson, B. (1984) *Making an Issue of Child Abuse. Political Agenda Setting for Social Problems.* Chicago: University of Chicago Press.
Nguyen, V-K. (2009) 'Government-by-exception: Enrolment and Experimentality in Mass HIV Treatment Programmes in Africa', *Social Theory & Health* 7, 196–217.
Ofri, D. (2009) 'The Emotional Epidemiology of H1N1 Influenza Vaccination', *New England Journal of Medicine* 361, 2594–2595.
Packard, R. (1989) *White Plague, Black Labor. Tuberculosis and the Political Economy of Health and Disease in South Africa.* Berkeley: University of California Press.
Petryna, A. (2002) *Life Exposed. Biological Citizens after Chernobyl.* Princeton, NJ: Princeton University Press.
Redfield, P. (2013) *Life In Crisis. The Ethical Journey of Doctors Without Borders.* Berkeley: University of California Press.
Scheper-Hughes, N. (2000) 'The Global Traffic in Human Organs', *Current Anthropology* 41 (2), 191–224.

Scott, J. (1985) *Weapons of the Weak. Everyday Forms of Peasant Resistance*. New Haven: Yale University Press.

Swanson, M. (1977) 'The Sanitation Syndrome: Bubonic Plague and Urban Native Policy in the Cape Colony, 1900–1909', *Journal of African History* 18 (3), 387–410.

Young, A. (1997) *The Harmony of Illusions. Inventing Post-Traumatic Stress Disorder*. Princeton, NJ: Princeton University Press.

Index

Accra Lunatic Asylum (Ghana) 112–114
Act-Up 237
acupuncture 15, 130–153
Africa 3–5, 10–11, 17, 81, 89–90, 99, 111, 113–116, 119–120, 124n.6, 154–155, 170–171, 176, 207–208, 217, 221–223, 230, 234–235
African Genome Variation Project 154
Alma Ata (conference, strategy) 6, 14, 62, 115
Almeida, Joel 67–68
Amrith, Sunil 6, 55
anatomy 141, 143
ancestry, genetic: 168–170, 173–175, 192, 201n.4
antibiotic(s) 8, 54, 60, 66
archive(s) 53, 60–61, 67–68, 70, 73, 75, 123n.2
Aro Mental Hospital (Nigeria) 85–87, 90, 93–94
Asare, Joseph 116–117
Asia 108, 130–131, 133–136, 139, 170–171, 176
association studies 164–168, 172–175
Asuni, Tolani 84–89, 95
Australia 137–138, 145
avian flu 242

Banerji, Debaber 33, 37, 66, 70–74
Barnett, Michael 238
Basaglia, Franco 107
BCG (Bacille Calmette-Guérin) 8, 54
Belgium 85
Bibeau, Gilles 234
Bill and Melinda Gates Foundation 1, 4, 233
Birn, Anne-Emanuelle 3, 21
Bolivia 35, 48
Botswana 3, 238
Brazil 17–18, 183–184, 190–200, 201n.4, 201n.5, 201n.10, 237
Brimnes, Nils 10, 55, 66, 73
Brown, Theodore 2–3, 225, 233
Brundtland, Gro Harlem 214–215, 218–19
Bryder, Lynda 54–55

cancer 1, 3, 17, 160, 164, 184, 186, 188, 190–199, 201n.4, 201n.5, 202n.10, 220, 231
  cancer genetics 186, 190–193, 199, 201n.4, 201n.5, 202n.10
  see also genetics
cardiovascular disease 1, 184
Carothers, John Colin 11, 90–91, 113–134
case-control studies: 172–175
Cassier, Maurice 7, 237
Centers for Disease Control (CDC) (US) 225n.1, 231–232
Centre d'Etude du Polymorphisme Humain (CEPH) (France) 163, 167, 170
Chabrol, Fanny 239
Chan, Margaret 208–210, 219, 221–224
chemotherapy(ies) 8–9, 54–56, 62, 65, 75n.3
Chen, Ken 140
Chikungunya 14
China 13, 56, 59, 65, 130, 132–137, 142, 210, 237, 242
Choi, Seung-hoon 140–146, 149n.15
clinic 18, 33, 36, 59, 67, 106, 117, 122, 124n.3, 147, 187, 190–192, 195, 199, 201n.4, 208, 223
clinical 5–6, 12, 15–18, 54, 58, 65, 74, 84, 87–89, 93, 131, 137, 140, 143, 157, 164, 185–195, 198–200, 209, 231, 235–236, 239–241
Cold War 3, 6
Collier, Stephen 105
colonial 4, 10–11, 60, 65, 72, 81–85, 87–93, 97–99, 105–106, 111–114, 120–122, 123n.3, 124n.4, 185, 236, 239
  see also colony(ies); post-colonial

colonialism 81–83, 89, 113, 169–170, 177
colonization 2
  see also decolonization
colony(ies) 5, 11, 106, 111–113, 124n.4
  see also colonial
Commission on Macroeconomics and Health (CMH) 215–216
Convention of the Rights of Persons with Disabilities (CRPD) 110, 117
cost-effectiveness 20, 216–217
Crane, Joanna 45–46
Crofton, John 63
Cunyngham-Brown, Robert 90, 111–113

data 12, 16, 29, 36, 44–45, 60, 63, 69, 72–74, 93–95, 98, 163, 167–170, 176, 186, 191, 194, 208, 238
Debata, Akio 138
decolonization 6, 83, 87, 99n.1
  see also colonization
deinstitutionalization 107–108, 111
depression 12, 92, 201n.3
development 1–3, 5–7, 11, 14, 22, 30, 55–56, 69–74, 76n.17, 82, 85–89, 98, 104, 107, 110, 122–123, 140, 157, 162, 167, 175–177, 187, 190, 195, 211, 215–217, 233, 236, 242
Dholakia, Ravindra H. 67–70, 73–74
Diagnostic and Statistical Manual (DSM) 10
Directly Observed Therapy, Short-Course (DOTS) 9, 38, 52
Directly Observed Treatment (DOT) 38, 39, 43, 44

Index

diversity (genetic) 154, 161, 167–170
DNA Polymorphism Discovery Resource 168–170
DNA sequencing 166
drug(s) 1, 4–9, 15, 20–21, 29–46, 52, 55–59, 63–67, 72–74, 87–88, 118–120, 167, 189, 200, 201n.3, 234–241
   resistance 21, 29–30, 33, 37, 39–41, 46, 55, 58, 64
   see also pharmaceuticals
Drugs for Neglected Diseases Initiative 218
Dubos, René J. 54

Ebola 207–213, 218–225, 226n.8, 230–232
economics 70, 74–75
   health economics 68, 70–71
epidemiology 7, 11, 22, 63–66, 70, 95, 165, 173, 183, 231
ethnography 56, 59–60, 122, 242
Europe 5–6, 13, 86, 95–96, 113–114, 123n.3, 130, 154–155, 161, 166, 170, 176, 183–188, 196, 241
European 2, 15, 54, 81–84, 90–94, 98, 108, 113, 123n.2, 131, 137, 156, 167, 176–177, 238
   European Commission 188
evolution (human): 158–161, 169

Fanon, Frantz 82
Farge, Arlette 53
Ferguson, James 235
Fischer, Walter 131, 145
Forster, Emmanuel 112–115, 118, 124n.5
Freud, Sigmund 85
Fujimura, Joan 175–176

Fukuda, Keiji 207
Furth, Charlotte 132

GAVI Alliance 218, 223
genetics 1, 8, 10, 15–18, 22, 154–161, 164–165, 170, 173, 176, 185–187, 190–193, 199, 201n.4, 201n.5, 202n.10
   cancer genetics 186, 190–193, 199, 201n4, 201n.5, 202n.10
   medical genetics 1, 8, 15–17, 22, 155, 164
genomics 15–18, 183–188, 198, 201n.4
Georgia 56, 59–60
Ghana 12–13, 103–106, 109–123, 123n.2, 124n.5
   see also Gold Coast
Giles-Vernick, Tamara 81
Global Burden of Disease (GBD) 7, 11–12, 16, 64, 70, 108–109
Global Fund to Fight AIDS, Tuberculosis and Malaria 217, 222, 226n.10
global history 82–83, 99
Glover, Susan 242
Gold Coast 111–112
   see also Ghana
guideline(s) 12, 29–30, 34, 39–46, 110, 140, 191, 240
Guinea 207–209, 230

Haiti 35, 56
Harper, Ian 10, 35–40, 56–58, 76n.17, 158
Harvard Medical School 230
health
   financing 71, 115
   governance of 1–2
   organization 225
      see also World Health Organization

research 82, 98, 109
system 33–39, 44–45, 71–73, 98, 115–119, 176, 190, 200, 222–223, 230
see also mental health
Hereditary Disease Foundation (HDF) 162
HIV 4, 8–9, 36, 55–57, 61, 65, 74, 81, 217, 234–242
Holm, Johannes 72
Hong Kong 138
Hsu, Elisabeth 132
Huang, Longxiang 144
Human Genome Diversity Project 154, 169–170
human rights 12–13, 22, 39, 103–111, 117–122,
Human Rights Watch (HRW) 13, 104–105, 117–118, 122

India 10, 13–15, 29–36, 40–46, 53–62, 66–75, 99n.4, 105, 109, 121, 131, 237
infectious disease(s) 7–8, 11, 54, 184
injuries 1
insecticide 5, 222
Instituto Nacional de Cancer (INCA) (Brazil) 190–191
International Haplotype Mapping (HapMap) Project 154, 170–171, 174–176
International Monetary Fund (IMF) 211, 215, 219
International Pilot Study of Schizophrenia (IPSS) 94–98
International Union Against Tuberculosis and Lung Disease (IUATLD) 9–10, 52–56, 61–65, 75n.5

Janes, Craig 233
Japan 96, 134, 137–146, 148n.10, 149n.17, 176, 242
Jawaharlal Nehru University (New Delhi) 70
judicialization (of health) 199–200

Kasolo, Francis 209
Kenya 92, 90, 176
Kilroy-Marac, Katie 105–106, 111, 124n.3
Koch, Erin 31, 56–60, 73
Korea 133–134, 137–146, 149n.17
Kyoto University (Japan) 137

Lachenal, Guillaume 4, 239
Lambo, Thomas A. 82–98, 114–115, 124n.5
Lander, Eric 164–167, 173
Latin America 13, 108, 215
Latour, Bruno 135, 147
Lei, Sean Hsiang-lin 133
Liberia 207, 230
Li-Fraumeni syndrome 192–200
Liu, Lydia 135, 139–142
Livingstone, Julie 238
localization 8, 21, 29–31, 42, 57, 98, 198
Lock, Margaret 10, 30, 131–132, 242

Ma, Eunjeong 133
MacFarlane, Sarah 233
Madras drug trials 55
Mahler, Halfdan 62, 66, 72
malaria 4–5, 8, 20, 67, 160, 217, 222
Malawi 53
Manuwa, Samuel 84
Massachusetts Institute of Technology (MIT) (US) 167, 243
Mbembe, Achille 106

Index

McGill University (Canada) 95–97
McMillen, Christian 8, 55
Mead, Margaret 85
Médecins sans Frontières (MSF) 36, 208, 237
Medical Research Council (MRC) 55–56, 62–63, 66, 74
medicinal herbs 131
mental
   disorder(s) 7, 10, 89, 108–110, 116, 119
   health 8, 10–13, 22, 81–84, 89, 98–99, 103–110, 113–123
   health care 82, 103–108, 113–122
   illness(es) 7, 11, 22, 82, 85, 89–90, 97–98, 104–111, 114–115, 119–121, 124n.3
Merry, Sally E. 104–105, 120
Metrics 1, 7, 11–12, 21, 45, 64, 109
Moulin, Anne-Marie 239
Mozambique 53
multi-drug resistant tuberculosis (MDR-TB) 29–46, 55
Murray, Christopher 7, 12, 32, 64–66

Nabarro, David 217
Nakajima, Hiroshi 214
Nakatani, Yoshio 137, 148n.9
National Institutes of Health (US) 170, 239
National Redemption Council (NRC) (Ghana) 115–116
National TB and Leprosy Program (NTLP) 61, 64–66, 75n.5
National Tuberculosis Institute (NTP) (Bengalore, India) 66–67, 70–73
nationalism 83, 89, 135
Needham, Joseph 130–131, 134, 147n.3

neglected disease 7–9, 201n.1, 218, 238
neoliberal 3, 6, 14, 19, 59–60, 122, 209, 211–219, 224, 226n.8, 236
neoliberalism 19, 211, 216
Nepal 35–36, 56–57
New Zealand 138
NGOs 4, 7, 44, 108, 116–117, 120, 218, 230, 237–238
Nguyen, Vinh-Kim 10, 30, 132, 235
Nigeria 11, 81–95, 98–99, 109, 124n.5, 170, 241
Nogier, Paul 131–133
nomenclature 134–140, 148n.11
non-communicable disease(s) 1, 7–8, 220

obesity 7
Ogden, Jessica 34, 38–39, 53, 56, 67
Oman 17
oncology 3, 186, 238

Packard, Randall 3, 7–8, 53, 217
patent(s) 15, 195, 217, 236
patient organizations 184, 188–189, 194
periodization 2, 5, 60
Peru 56, 238
Petryna, Adriana 7, 30, 202n.7, 239
pharmaceutical(s) 12, 14–15, 29, 75, 187
pharmaceutical
   companies 4, 167, 237
   industry 6, 200, 236
   firms 210
   see also drug(s)
philanthropy 1
Philippines (the) 14, 137–138

population(s) 1, 6, 16–19, 29, 63, 66, 84, 88–90, 109, 119, 154–161, 167–176, 183–184, 186–196, 201n.4, 201n.5, 213, 217, 234–241
population isolates 160–161, 166, 169
post-colonial 11, 72, 81–8 2, 99, 105, 122, 124n.4, 185, 236
　see also colonial
Post-Traumatic Stress Disorder (PTSD) 12, 237
poverty 1, 9, 34–37, 215–216, 238
President's Emergency Plan for AIDS Relief (PEPFAR) 235
primary health care (PHC) 1, 12, 17–21, 59, 62, 67, 72
Pritzker, Sonya E. 135
protocol(s) 10, 30, 45, 62–64, 191–192, 235
psychiatric hospital 84, 103, 108–109, 112, 115–121
　see also psychiatry
psychiatrist 84, 94, 114, 117, 124n.5
　see also psychiatry
psychiatry 10–12, 81–91, 98, 105–110, 113–116, 119, 124n.4, 124n.5
　colonial 83, 89, 113
　cross-cultural 81, 94
　　see also psychiatric hospital; psychiatrist
public health 2–8, 11, 14, 16–17, 30, 33, 35, 38–41, 46, 54, 66, 71, 81, 88, 131, 183–193, 200, 201n.4, 202n.7, 209, 213, 216, 222–225, 233, 237–239
public health emergency 208
public-private partnerships 1, 3–4, 7, 20, 167, 217–220

race 18, 92, 158–159, 171, 175–176, 185
Redfield, Peter 238
Revised National Tuberculosis Control Programme (RNTCP) (India) 32–34, 38–41, 44–47, 66–67
risk(s) 7–9, 17, 20, 30, 38, 43–45, 139, 160, 164–165, 174, 190–196, 199, 201n.4, 231–232, 235
Rouillon, Anick 75n.6
Russia 56
Ryan, Frank 55

Sanatorium (as sanatoria) 4
SARS 14, 218–219
Scheid, Volker 132
Scheper-Hughes, Nancy 107, 237
Schiebinger, Londa 147
schizophrenia 88–98
Scott, James 236
Seeberg, Jens 33, 37–38, 56–58
Senegal 43, 89, 106, 124n.3, 124n.4, 124n.5
Sierra Leone 207, 230
Singapore 138, 145
Sismondo, Sergio 136, 145
smallpox 5, 210, 218
Smith, Francis B. 54
SNP Consortium 167–170
Soulie de Morant, George 131
South Africa 56–58, 116, 237, 240–241
sputum microscopy 31–32, 63
standard(s) 10, 29–30, 37, 40, 44–46, 57, 63, 66–67, 104, 107, 119, 120, 134–147, 148n.12, 149n.21, 150n.22

Index

standardization 5, 7, 10, 29–31, 36–42, 45–46, 57, 134–138, 141, 145
Stiefvater, Eric H. W. 131
structural adjustment 4, 19, 59, 115
Styblo, Karel 61–66, 76n.10
support
    nutritional 40, 43–44
    social 44
Swanson, Maynard 241
Swedish International Development Agency (SIDA) 70
swine flu 210, 242

Tanzania 4, 10, 52–55, 59–66, 75, 89
Third World (the) 6, 63, 238–239
Trade-Related Aspects of Intellectual Property Rights (TRIPS) 15, 236
traditional
    Chinese medicine (TCM) 130–135, 139, 142, 145
    medicine 8, 13–14, 131–133, 140
    healing 4, 109, 111, 124n.5
Tsutani, Kiichiro 139, 148n.12
tuberculosis (TB) 3, 7–10, 20–22, 29–46, 52–75, 62–63, 66, 70, 217, 240–241

UK (the) 84, 105, 108, 113, 116, 119–120, 137, 145, 167, 187–189, 211
UNAIDS 238–240
United Nations (UN) 3, 5, 8, 13, 89, 105–110, 116–122, 137–138, 207, 213, 217–218, 224
United States (US) 5–6, 13–15, 86, 96, 107–108, 116, 121, 123n.3, 130–131, 133, 137, 145, 163,167, 170, 185–197, 211–214, 230–239
University of California, Los Angeles (UCLA) 239
University of Ibadan (Nigeria) 87
Unschuld, Paul 139, 145

vaccine(s) 5, 54–55, 196, 218, 223
variation (genetic) 154, 158–160, 167–169, 171–172, 176–177, 186
Victoriaborg Castle (Ghana) 112
Vietnam 138–139, 145
voluntary donations 221

Wang, Deshen 133
Webb, James 6, 81
Wexler, Milton 162
Wiseman, Nigel 142
Wittgenstein, Ludwig 146
World Bank (the) 3, 7–10, 19–20, 31–32, 52–53, 57–60, 64–71, 76n.16, 108, 115–116, 211–216, 219,224
World Health Assembly (of WHO) 14, 208, 212–214, 223
World Health Organization (WHO) 3–6, 9–20, 31–34, 38–39, 42–43, 52–53, 57, 60–62, 65–70, 75n.1, 81, 87–89, 94–97, 104–110, 115–116, 120–122, 123n.2, 131, 134–140, 143–146, 148n.12, 185, 188, 207–225, 225n.1, 230–233, 241
World Trade Organization (WTO) 215–217, 236

Yaba Lunatic Asylum (Nigeria) 84
Young, Allan 12, 237

EU authorised representative for GPSR:
Easy Access System Europe, Mustamäe tee 50,
10621 Tallinn, Estonia
gpsr.requests@easproject.com

www.ingramcontent.com/pod-product-compliance
Ingram Content Group UK Ltd.
Pitfield, Milton Keynes, MK11 3LW, UK
UKHW021830210426
5322IPUK00004B/122